CHEMOTHERAPY OF GYNECOLOGIC CANCERS:

Society of Gynecologic Oncologists Handbook, 2e

D1081799

CHEMOTHERAPY OF GYNECOLOGIC CANCERS:

Society of Gynecologic Oncologists Handbook, 2e

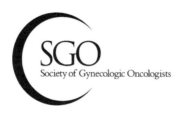

EDITED BY

STEPHEN C. RUBIN, MD

Professor and Director
Division of Gynecologic Oncology
University of Pennsylvania Medical Center
Philadelphia, Pennsylvania

WITH 16 CONTRIBUTORS

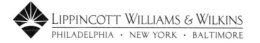

LIPPINCOTT WILLIAMS & WILKINS
PHILADELPHIA · NEW YORK · BALTIMORE

Acquisitions Editor: Jonathan Pine
Developmental Editor: Erin McMullan
Production Manager: Jennifer Jett
Cover Designer: Lou Moriconi
Compositor: Maryland Composition, Inc.
Printer/Binder: Transcontinental Printing

Copyright © 2004 Society of Gynecologic Oncologists

351 West Camden Street
Baltimore, Maryland 21201-2436 USA

530 Walnut Street
Philadelphia, PA 19106

All rights reserved. This book is protected by copyright. No part of this book may be reproduced in any form or by any means, including photocopying, or utilized by any information storage and retrieval system without written permission from the copyright owner.

The publisher is not responsible (as a matter of product liability, negligence, or otherwise) for any injury resulting from any material contained herein. This publication contains information relating to general principles of medical care that should not be construed as specific instructions for individual patients. Manufacturers' product information and package inserts should be reviewed for current information; including contraindications, dosages, and precautions.

Printed in Canada

Library of Congress Cataloging-in-Publication Data

ISBN: 0-7817-4891-7

The publishers have made every effort to trace the copyright holders for borrowed material. If they have inadvertently overlooked any, they will be pleased to make the necessary arrangements at the first opportunity.

To purchase additional copies of this book, call our customer service department at **(800) 638-3030** or fax orders to **(301) 824-7390**. International customers should call **(301) 714-2324**.

Visit Lippincott Williams & Wilkins on the Internet: http://www.LWW.com. Lippincott Williams & Wilkins customer service representatives are available from 8:30 am to 6:00 pm, EST.

03 04 05 06 07

1 2 3 4 5 6 7 8 9 10

— *DEDICATION* —

To Anne, Mike, and Ellie

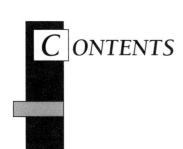

CONTENTS

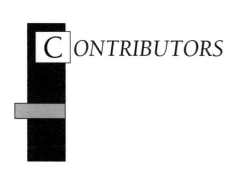

CONTRIBUTORS

JEFFREY E. BALL, MD
Fellow
Hematology-Oncology
Temple/Fox Chase Cancer Center
Philadelphia, Pennsylvania

RICHARD R. BARAKAT, MD
Chief, Gynecology Service
Department of Surgery
Memorial Sloan-Kettering Cancer Institute
New York, New York
Associate Professor
Department of Obstetrics and Gynecology
Weill Medical College of Cornell University
New York, New York

IVOR BENJAMIN, MD
Digital Ingenuity
Philadelphia, Pennsylvania

JOHN BLESSING, MD
GOG Statistical & Data Center
Roswell Park Cancer Institute
Buffalo, New York

CHRISTINA S. CHU, MD
Assistant Professor
Department of Obstetrics and Gynecology
Division of Gynecologic Oncology
University of Pennsylvania School of Medicine
Philadelphia, Pennsylvania

JOHN P. CURTIN, MD
Professor and Chair
Department of Obstetrics and Gynecology
Director, Gynecologic Oncology
New York University School of Medicine
New York, New York

JAKOB DUPONT, MD
Clinical Assistant Professor
Department of Medicine
Memorial Sloan-Kettering Cancer Institute
New York, New York
Instructor
Department of Medicine
Weill Medical College of Cornell University
New York, New York

MAURIE MARKMAN, MD
Chairman
Department of Hematology/Medical Oncology
The Cleveland Clinic Foundation
Cleveland, Ohio

ANDREW W. MENZIN, MD
Clinical Associate Professor
Department of Obstetrics and Gynecology
New York University School of Medicine
New York, New York
Associate Chief, Gynecologic Oncology
Department of Obstetrics and Gynecology
North Shore University Hospital
Manhasset, New York

MARK A. MORGAN, MD
Associate Professor
Department of Obstetrics and Gynecology
Division of Gynecologic Oncology
University of Pennsylvania School of Medicine
Philadelphia, Pennsylvania

THOMAS P. MORRISSEY, MD
Assistant Professor
Department of Obstetrics and Gynecology
New York University School of Medicine
New York, New York
Attending Surgeon
Department of Gynecologic Oncology
North Shore University Hospital
Manhasset, New York

RUSSELL J. SCHILDER, MD
Member
Medical Oncology
Fox Chase Cancer Center
Philadelphia, Pennsylvania
Associate Professor
Department of Medicine
Temple University School of Medicine
Philadelphia, Pennsylvania

YUKIO SONODA, MD
Assistant Attending Surgeon
Department of Surgery, Gynecology Service
Memorial Sloan-Kettering Cancer Institute
New York, New York
Assistant Professor
Department of Obstetrics and Gynecology
Weill Medical College of Cornell University
New York, New York

MIKA A. SOVAK, MD, PHD
Medical Oncology Fellow
Department of Medicine
Memorial Sloan-Kettering Cancer Institute
New York, New York

DAVID SPRIGGS
Chief, Developmental Chemotherapy
Department of Medicine
Memorial Sloan-Kettering Cancer Institute
New York, New York

J. TATE THIGPEN, MD
Professor of Medicine
Director, Division of Oncology
Department of Medicine
University of Mississippi School of Medicine
Jackson, Mississippi

PREFACE TO THE SECOND EDITION

Considerable progress has been made in the chemotherapy of gynecologic cancers since the first edition of this text. Carboplatin and paclitaxel are now a part of the standard treatment for ovarian cancer, the activity of several newer agents against ovarian cancer has been documented in the second-line setting, and trials of these agents in the primary disease setting are underway. New information has emerged regarding the role of chemotherapy in endometrial cancer, and chemotherapy combined with radiation therapy is now the standard of care in many patients with cervical cancer. Similarly, much progress has been made in ameliorating the side effects and complications of chemotherapy. New dosing regimens, new cytokines, new antiemetics, and new antibiotics are among the improvements.

These advances, and much more, have been chronicled in the second edition of the *Chemotherapy of Gynecologic Cancers: Society of Gynecologic Oncologists Handbook,* which again has brought together an outstanding assortment of leading experts in the field to author concise, clinically relevant chapters that will be of value to practitioners in their day-to-day care of women with gynecologic cancer.

PREFACE TO THE FIRST EDITION

Gynecologic cancers are among the leading causes of cancer death in women. Over the last 20 years, remarkable advances have been made in the chemotherapy of these malignancies, including the development of new cytotoxic drugs, the refinement of combination chemotherapy regimens, and the introduction of new methods to minimize and treat chemotherapy toxicity. These advances have led to major improvements in outcome for women with gynecologic cancers. Despite this proliferation of knowledge about the chemotherapy of gynecologic cancers, until this time there has been no single text that brings together in a highly structured, concise, clinically relevant format the material needed by clinicians as they care for gynecologic cancer patients undergoing chemotherapy. This book was developed by the Society of Gynecologic Oncologists to fill that void.

The book brings together recognized experts from the fields of gynecologic oncology and medical oncology to provide a comprehensive yet practical overview of all aspects of the chemotherapy of gynecologic cancers. The book opens with chapters on the basic principles of chemotherapy, and the clinical pharmacology, mechanisms of action, and toxicities of the drugs used in the treatment of gynecologic malignancies. Subsequent chapters deal with the design of clinical trials and with the specific chemotherapy of gynecologic cancers by site and stage. The use of intraperitoneal chemotherapy is considered in detail. Later chapters deal with practical issues such as central venous catheters, premedication of the chemotherapy patient, management of chemotherapy complications, and the use of blood products and growth factors.

Chemotherapy of Gynecologic Cancers: Society of Gynecologic Oncologists Handbook is intended to provide both the experienced practitioner and the trainee with a thorough, succinct reference that will be of use in their day-to-day practice. Its success will be measured by the extent to which it helps us in our common goal: improving the care of women with gynecologic cancer.

ACKNOWLEDGMENTS

The Society of Gynecologic Oncologists gratefully acknowledges a generous educational grant from Bristol-Myers Squibb Oncology in support of the development and distribution of this handbook.

The editor would like to acknowledge Carmen Lord, Editorial Assistant in the Division of Gynecologic Oncology at the University of Pennsylvania, Jonathan W. Pine, Jr., Senior Executive Editor at Lippincott Williams & Wilkins, and the individual authors of the chapters herein, whose efforts made the second edition of this text possible.

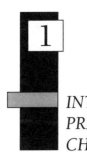

INTRODUCTION AND PRINCIPLES OF CHEMOTHERAPY

JEFFREY E. BALL AND RUSSELL J. SCHILDER

Brief History of the Development of Cancer Chemotherapy

Although occasional reports of the anticancer effects of drugs appeared more than 100 years ago, cancer chemotherapy as we know it today began in the 1940s with a series of developments, including the publication of the Nobel Prize-winning work on the antitumor effect of estrogens in prostate cancer. In the same decade, the war effort produced nitrogen mustard, one of a series of alkylating agents (a class of compounds) that continues to find utility as part of many combination chemotherapy regimens. Between 1945 and 1965, a wide variety of active chemotherapeutic agents were identified and developed, including actinomycin D, the vinca alkaloids, fluorouracil (5-FU), progesterones, and cyclophosphamide. In the early 1970s, cisplatin was shown to have significant activity in ovarian and testicular cancer, and doxorubicin, bleomycin, and the epipodophyllotoxins (VP-16 and VM-26) became available for clinical use. During the same decade, tamoxifen was shown to have significant activity in breast cancer as treatment in the adjuvant setting and for advanced disease. In the 1980s and 1990s, agents with activity in ovarian and breast cancer, such as ifosfamide (with mesna) and paclitaxel, were introduced into general prac-

Chemotherapy of Gynecologic Cancers: Society of Gynecologic Oncologists Handbook 2e, edited by Stephen C. Rubin, MD, Lippincott Williams & Wilkins, Philadelphia © 2004.

tice. More recent developments include the introduction of useful derivatives of parent compounds, such as carboplatin, idarubicin, and docetaxel. Newer compounds, such as the topoisomerase I inhibitors (topotecan and irinotecan), as well as monoclonal antibodies directed against cell-surface components, such as trastuzumab (Herceptin), have ushered in the era of molecular-targeted therapies.

The use of biological agents in the treatment of cancer began in the 1960s and has accelerated to the present day. These applications have included the use of monoclonal antibodies for both diagnostic and therapeutic purposes, the use of interferons, and the application of hematopoietic growth factors such as erythropoietin and the colony stimulating factors (sargramostim and filgrastim), which have reduced hematopoietic side effects and allowed the exploration of increased dose intensity.

For the foreseeable future, we can expect an expansion of chemotherapeutic agents specifically designed for a variety of molecular targets emerging from knowledge of molecular oncology, as typified by imatinib mesylate (Gleevec) and gefitinib (Iressa).

■■■ Cell Cycle and Growth Kinetics

Many of the principles of chemotherapy have been derived from knowledge about the growth patterns of normal and neoplastic tissues. Differences in the growth characteristics of different tissues have contributed to particular strategies of chemotherapy use and have also contributed substantially to our understanding of the toxicities produced by chemotherapeutic agents.

Normal tissues can be divided broadly into three categories: static, expanding, and renewing. Static populations of well-differentiated cells rarely undergo cell division and are not actively proliferating during most of adult life. Tissues such as striated muscle and nerve tissue are examples of static populations. These tissues are ordinarily not affected by drugs that work on rapidly proliferating cells.

Expanding populations usually do not proliferate rapidly, although they retain their capacity to do so when exposed to stress or injury. The liver is an example of an organ containing expanding cell populations. Renewing cell populations, the third type found in normal tissue, are constantly proliferating and renewing, and are in constant cell division. Examples include bone marrow and gastrointestinal mucosa. An understanding of these three broad types of normal tissue growth partially explains the toxicities associated with common chemotherapeutic agents targeting these cell populations. Static and expanding cell populations are generally less injured by chemotherapy, whereas renewing cell populations are commonly most affected by anticancer drugs.

The unregulated growth that is characteristic of cancer is associated with loss of the normal cell control mechanisms operative in noncancerous tissues. Despite the uncontrolled nature of this growth, studies indicate that cell division in cancer cells does not occur more rapidly when compared with division of normal cells. Increasing evidence indicates that loss of normal cell-cycle regulation and a failure of apoptosis (programmed cell death) are the primary reasons for this uncontrolled cell growth.

As tumors grow, they generally display what is known as Gompertzian growth, meaning that as tumor mass increases, the time required for the tumor mass to double also increases. This pattern of growth results in rapid initial proliferation, followed by a progressive increase in the doubling time of the tumor. Although at first glance this suggests that tumors should grow rapidly when they are small and then more slowly when they are large, clinically the opposite appears to occur. When tumors become palpable they are already large, and a small number of doublings results in a huge change in tumor size. Limited information is available on the doubling time of human tumors, but to the extent studied, doubling times vary greatly from about 1 month in certain embryonal tumors to as long as 6 months in certain adenocarcinomas.

Doubling times refer to the growth of an entire heterogeneous tumor mass, whereas the cell cycle generally refers to the activity of individual tumor cells. The cell cycle is divided into four phases. The first is the mitotic phase (M phase), the point of chromosomal division. The second phase is a variable period known as G_1 after cell division in which cellular activities, protein and RNA synthesis, and DNA repair occur. G_1 cells can terminally differentiate into what is known as G_0 or noncycling cells, or they can reenter the cell cycle after a period of quiescence. Following G_1 is the S phase, a period in which new DNA is synthesized. Finally, after the completion of DNA synthesis, the cell enters the G_2 period with twice the basal DNA content. The G_2 phase is ordinarily short, and the cell reenters mitosis and cell division occurs. Both normal and tumor cells are sensitive to many chemotherapeutic agents during the active cell-cycling period. Conversely, they are considerably less sensitive to chemotherapy during the resting or G_0 phase.

Cell cycle times may be determined by performing labeled mitosis studies in which labeling is used to mark the cell cycle during the S phase. The time between the subsequent waves of cell division defines the length of the cell cycle. From studies in human tumors, cell cycle times from 10 to 31 hours have been established and there is considerably less variation in cell cycle times than in previously mentioned tumor doubling times.

Chemotherapeutic agents have multiple mechanisms of action and affect tumor cells in various ways. Nevertheless, particular chemotherapeutic agents are known to be proliferation dependent and/or cell-cycle specific, like cytosine arabinoside or hydroxyurea. Other chemotherapeutic agents are cell-cycle nonspecific and less proliferation dependent, such as nitrogen mustard or actinomycin D. The differences in cell-cycle specificity and proliferation dependency often explain why certain combination strategies are utilized, combining both cell-cycle–specific with cell-cycle–nonspecific drugs and proliferation-dependent with proliferation-independent drugs.

In concepts derived from animal model data, the curability of cancers is inversely proportional to the number of viable tumor cells with the cancer, the so-called tumor burden. Therefore, treatment applied when the tumor is subclinical in size results in more cures than when the tumor is large, and this kinetic concept has led to the use of adjuvant chemotherapy in patients with potentially curable diseases at high risk or recurrence. First-order kinetics is another concept derived from animal tumor models in which chemotherapeutic agents have been shown to kill a constant *fraction* of cells exposed to the drug, rather than a constant number. This has led to the use of multiple cycles of therapy rather than the one-time administration of chemotherapeutic agents. Understanding the kinetic alterations produced by cytotoxic drugs and the cellular kinetics of normal and neoplastic tissues has provided the physician with a more scientific basis for the application of single drugs or drugs in combination.

Pharmacologic Principles

The specific chemotherapeutic agents used in the treatment of gynecologic malignancies will be covered in other chapters in this book. However, there are a variety of characteristics that determine the appropriate use of particular anticancer drugs either alone or in combination. These factors include the mechanism of action, absorption, distribution, metabolism, and excretion of the particular chemotherapeutic agent. These properties not only influence drug effectiveness *in vivo*, but they provide additional rationale for the selection of drugs for use in combination. The different routes of administration also influence drug selection and patient acceptability. Drugs may be administered orally, intravenously, intramuscularly, intraarterially, or intraperitoneally, and the selection of the route of administration depends on the feasibility, patient acceptance, and potential for toxicity of the agents selected. The route of administration can also affect the optimal *concentration x time* calculation, also known as the area under the curve (AUC), on which drug effectiveness is at least partially dependent. Ultimately, the effectiveness of a particular chemotherapeutic agent is in part a function of the concentration of the active drug moiety and the duration of exposure at the critical tumor sites.

Because the AUC of the active agent at tumor sites determines, in part, the effectiveness of a given drug, the distribution and transport of a chemotherapeutic agent can influence this calculation. Binding of the drug to serum albumin or to plastic catheters can alter active drug concentrations. The lipid solubility or the membrane transport also may substantially alter the concentration of drug delivered to critical tissue sites. Some areas of the body, such as the brain or the testes, function as pharmacologic sanctuaries with impaired drug entry into these sites. Likewise, hypoxic areas within necrotic tumors may be poorly perfused with critical concentrations of drug. Certain drugs such as mitomycin C or 5-FU passively diffuse through cell membranes, whereas others such as cisplatin or melphalan require active carrier transport systems.

Many chemotherapeutic agents are active as intact drugs, but others like cyclophosphamide are prodrugs and require hepatic P-450 activation before producing any antitumor effects. Obviously, drugs requiring hepatic activation are ineffective when given via the intraperitoneal or intraarterial routes because direct delivery of high concentrations of prodrugs produce no therapeutic advantage.

The biologically active drug AUC will also be substantially affected by drug metabolism including inactivation, elimination, or excretion. The two primary sites of inactivation and excretion of most chemotherapeutic agents are the liver and kidneys, respectively, although minor excretion also may occur through the stool and through respiration. Hepatic or renal dysfunction resulting from prior chemotherapy, underlying disease, or other drug-related toxicities may seriously impair drug excretion and correspondingly increase drug toxicity. Doses of doxorubicin or vincristine may require modification if there is significant underlying liver disease because these drugs are primarily excreted in the bile. Impaired renal function may seriously increase toxicity from cisplatin, carboplatin, and etoposide.

All of the previously discussed factors are considered when calculating the dose of a chemotherapeutic agent. Most chemotherapeutic agents have a narrow therapeutic range. After selecting a drug or a combination of drugs to be given to a patient, the dose must be calculated accurately in order to achieve an optimal AUC and to avoid undue toxicity. Some chemotherapeutic agents are dosed on a mg/kg basis (prednisone, busulfan), but most doses are calculated taking into account a patient's height and weight, using body surface area (mg/m^2). This modification normalizes for body frame and ensures that each patient receives proportionally the same amount of drug. A more recent dosing strategy (the Calvert formula) used for carboplatin incorporates pharmacokinetic principles directly into the dosage calculation. The Calvert formula acknowledges that myelosuppression especially thrombocytopenia, a major pharmacodynamic effect, is directly related to the degree of renal dysfunction, as reflected by the patient's glomerular filtration rate.

███ Drug Interactions

The average cancer patient receives a wide variety of drugs, including analgesics, antibiotics, and antiemetics, in addition to other common drugs used to control chronic diseases. Some of these drug interactions are particularly important and may substantially alter drug toxicity. Examples relevant to gynecologic cancer chemotherapy are the increased toxicity of doxorubicin and the taxanes (paclitaxel and docetaxel) in patients with impaired biliary excretion and the increased toxicity of cisplatin in patients with renal impairment; the displacement of methotrexate from plasma proteins by aspirin or sulfonamides; and the direct chemical interaction between mitoxantrone and heparin. The reader is referred to more detailed reviews of drug interactions for a more comprehensive discussion of the subject.

▮▮▮▮ Drug Resistance

One of the most frustrating aspects of cancer treatment is the tendency of many tumors to respond dramatically to initial treatment and then gradually become resistant to that treatment and all other subsequent treatments. Drug resistance may be intrinsic or acquired, and it may develop to one drug or to multiple agents. Intrinsic drug resistance is seen when tumors are first exposed to chemotherapeutic agents and fail to respond in any measurable way to initial therapy. Acquired drug resistance occurs when tumors no longer respond to drugs to which they were initially sensitive. Acquired resistance may be to a specific chemotherapeutic agent (i.e., methotrexate resistance caused by amplification of the dihydrofolate reductase gene), or it may be pleiotropic, meaning it is associated with resistance to multiple chemotherapeutic agents such as mediated through the mdr gene product.

There are a wide variety of mechanisms that determine specific drug resistance. These include defective drug transport, altered drug activation, altered hormone receptor concentration or affinity, altered DNA repair, gene amplification, altered target proteins, defective drug metabolism, and altered intracellular nucleotide pools. Examples relevant to gynecologic malignancies include altered hormone receptor concentrations or altered binding associated with resistance to steroid hormone therapy; enhanced DNA repair and increased removal of platinum-associated adducts in cisplatin and carboplatin resistance; and a specific transport effect associated with low carrier-mediated uptake of melphalan.

Just as there are specific mechanisms of resistance important in cancer chemotherapy in general, there also are different mechanisms of multidrug resistance. The best characterized multidrug resistance mechanism is associated with *MDR1* gene and its protein product, the P170 glycoprotein. Upon exposure to natural products, some tumors develop cross-resistance to a variety of structurally unrelated chemotherapeutic agents derived from natural products. Resistance associated with this mechanism generally includes drugs like the vinca alkaloids, actinomycin D, doxorubicin, and paclitaxel. The P170 glycoprotein functions as a drug-efflux pump, lowering the intracellular concentrations of these drugs. This mechanism of multidrug resistance has been documented to occur in human ovarian cancer cells. Although the MDR1 mechanism of multidrug resistance is the best studied to date, it is clear that alternate forms of multidrug resistance exist. Tumor cell lines resistant to many, but not all, natural products that do not demonstrate the MDR1 phenotype have been described. Other mechanisms of multidrug resistance include increased intracellular glutathione concentrations, which confers resistance to alkylating agents and radiation therapy. In addition, there are a variety of resistance mechanisms related to genes controlling either growth arrest or apoptosis (programmed cell death). It is likely that a wide variety of drug resistance mechanisms develop *in vivo*, and that admixtures of these mechanisms produce the spectrum of drug resistance that is seen clinically.

████ *Dose Intensity*

The successful use of drug therapy in cancer treatment usually has required the appropriate selection of an active drug or drugs in combination. It also is clear that the intensity with which the drugs are administered has an important influence on successful treatment. It has long been known from the successful treatment of choriocarcinoma, testicular cancers, and other germ cell tumors that inadequate doses of active treatment are not curative. In contrast, full doses of active regimens are associated with optimal outcomes. Likewise, evidence from the cures produced with high-dose-intensity regimens associated with hematopoietic stem cell support in diffuse large-cell lymphoma, acute leukemia, and

Hodgkin's lymphoma documents the clinical relevance of the concept of dose intensity.

Dose intensity is a measure of the amount of drug administered over time. Analysis requires that each drug regimen be converted to some standard, independent of the schedule of drug administration. The standard has typically been $mg/m^2/week$. After the dosage of an individual drug in any particular regimen has been expressed in $mg/m^2/week$, the regimen can be compared with the dose intensity of any other similar regimen.

Retrospective analysis of data on a large number of advanced breast cancer trials, advanced ovarian cancer trials, and lymphoma studies documented the importance of the dose-intensity concept. In many of these retrospective studies, there was a linear relationship between dose intensity and outcome. In the retrospective analysis done in advanced ovarian cancer, the dose intensity of compared regimens correlated well with outcome. In these trials, the dose-intensity effect was most important for cisplatin and any other two-drug combination, but did not appear to be correlated for most single-agent chemotherapy, particularly with alkylating agents.

Although most of the information demonstrating the importance of dose intensity has been retrospective, several prospective studies tend to support the concept. In a study comparing different levels of dose intensity of the breast cancer regimen CMF (cyclophosphamide, methotrexate, and fluorouracil), the higher-dose-intensity regimen was associated with a substantial increase in response rate, consistent with the retrospectively generated data. In contrast, a well-done two-dose-intensity study of cisplatin-cyclophosphamide in advanced ovarian cancer by the Gynecologic Oncology Group failed to demonstrate a significant benefit from a dose-intensity regimen that almost doubled the dose intensity while leaving the total dose of chemotherapy constant.

It is likely that the importance of dose intensity is greatest in highly responsive tumors where cure can be achieved with chemotherapy. In that setting, high dose intensity maximizes those cure rates. In other less sensitive tumors, it may not be possible to increase the dose to a level sufficient to produce demonstrable benefit without producing dose-limiting toxicity. Thus far, trials utilizing higher-dose chemotherapy with peripheral blood stem cell support have not improved outcomes in patients with gynecologic malignancies. Nevertheless, it is evident that reducing dose intensity as a means of regulating toxicity produces inferior therapeutic results.

████ Principles of Combination Chemotherapy

Effective chemotherapy generally requires combinations of active agents to produce optimal antitumor effect. Combination chemotherapy is able to achieve results that are not easily accomplished with single drugs. Combinations generally can maximize cell kill by using several drugs with different toxicities in a way that allows the antitumor effect of the combination to be maximized without undue toxicities. Combination chemotherapy also is more likely to effectively attack heterogeneous populations of cells with different mechanisms of resistance that are characteristic of human tumors. The use of multiple drugs with different mechanisms of action tends to minimize the emergence of drug resistance. Drugs used in any combination should have clinical data indicating that their effects will be synergistic or at least additive. Despite some interesting animal data to the contrary, there is no evidence that individual drugs that are inactive in a particular human tumor can be made active by their use in combination. The effectiveness and tolerance of a particular combination are enhanced when drugs with different spectra of toxicity are used, so that overlapping toxicities do not become dose limiting. Drugs in combination should be used at their optimal doses and schedules; the practice of dose reduction to allow the addition of other agents is generally counterproductive. Drugs in combination should be administered intermittently to maximize cell kill, minimize immunosuppression, and allow hematopoietic recovery. It is valuable to keep the interval between courses as short as possible, to allow bone marrow and/or other target organ recovery but not allow equivalent recovery of the tumor when developing a treatment strategy.

It is instructive for the clinician to ask the following questions when evaluating any particular proposed drug combination:

1. Is combination chemotherapy the treatment of choice for that particular stage of disease?
2. How long has the regimen been in active use, and has activity been documented in more than 1 study?
3. Has the combination regimen been published in a way that allows adequate description of potential side effects?
4. Does the combination regimen contain unusual drugs or schedules that require special facilities or complex monitoring?
5. Does the combination include drugs that are commercially available or is it investigational with limited access through the National Cancer Institute or pharmaceutical company programs?

Generally, the answers to these five questions will allow most physicians to determine the potential utility of a particular drug combination in their patient.

Combination chemotherapy is used in a variety of different situations depending on the extent of disease present and the probability of recurrence. Treatment is referred to as *induction chemotherapy* when combinations are used as initial therapy for patients with disseminated disease. In contrast, *adjuvant chemotherapy* refers to the use of combinations after the primary tumor has been definitively treated, but the risk of recurrence is high. The term *neoadjuvant chemotherapy* is used when drug treatment is applied in the management of local disease before the use of surgery or radiation therapy, to decrease the extent or morbidity of the definitive regional treatment. Therapy applied after disease recurrence of if tumor proves refractory to initial induction treatment is often referred to as *salvage chemotherapy*.

▬▬ *Overview of Chemotherapy Toxicity*

As discussed earlier in this chapter, the brunt of chemotherapy toxicity is born by tissues undergoing rapid proliferation. In addition, there are sometimes unique target tissues that are unusually sensitive to particular chemotherapeutic agents. Bone marrow is the most common site for toxic side effects because of its rapid and its rapid and continuous regeneration. Leukopenia generally occurs 7 to 10 days after treatment and persists for 3 to 10 days, and patients are at increased risk for infectious complications during these periods. Thrombocytopenia also commonly occurs and is generally slightly delayed in both its onset and recovery compared to leukopenia. During periods when the platelet count is less than $50,000/mm^3$, and particularly when the platelet count is less than $10,000/mm^3$, patients are at increased risk for hemorrhagic complications. Serious bone marrow suppression can be partially corrected with the use of hematopoietic growth factors such as filgrastim or sargramostim, erythropoietin (or its analogue darbepoetin alfa), or oprelvekin.

Gastrointestinal toxicity also is frequently seen. Many drugs and regimens are associated with nausea and vomiting. Depending on the magnitude of the side effect, a series of progressively more potent antiemetic compounds may be administered to reduce this toxicity. In mild situations, nausea and vomiting can be effectively managed by prochlorperazine or dexamethasone. A $5\text{-}HT_3$ antagonist can be used, either alone or in combination with dexamethasone in more severe cases. In addition to nausea and vomiting, diarrhea, mucositis, and esophagitis can be difficult side effects to manage and occasionally dose limiting. Alopecia, while not life threatening, is one of the most disturbing and emotionally discouraging of all toxicities associated with chemotherapy, particularly for women. It is commonly associated with drugs such as cisplatin, cyclophosphamide, doxorubicin, and paclitaxel. Nevertheless, variable degrees of alopecia can occur with a variety of chemotherapeutic agents, and patients should be well informed about this potential toxicity in advance. The major neurotoxicity commonly encountered is peripheral neuropathy, which occurs with the administration of cisplatin, taxanes, altretamine, and the vinca alkaloids. Most troublesome is the cisplatin-induced neurotoxicity that is usually sensory in type and delayed in onset. Progression of this type of neurotoxicity can occur after the completion of drug therapy and is very slow to resolve. Other neurotoxicities induced by chemotherapy include acute cerebellar syndromes, cranial nerve palsies or paralysis, and occasionally acute and chronic encephalopathies.

Genitourinary toxicity generally affects the kidneys or urinary bladder. Cisplatin therapy frequently results in renal dysfunction if appropriate urinary output before and after therapy is not maintained. Admixture of cisplatin with mannitol in normal saline, along with the use of loop diuretics, decreases the risk of causing renal injury. Hemorrhagic cystitis can be seen in patients treated with cyclophosphamide, or particularly ifosfamide, although this complication can be prevented by maintaining high urinary output and simultaneously administering mesna (a sulfhydryl-group donor), especially with the ifosfamide.

Skin toxicities encompass a wide variety of complications. Changes in skin pigmentation are seen with bleomycin and 5-FU; nail discoloration and oncholysis have been associated with docetaxel therapy. Extravasation necrosis is a serious complication seen with several frequently used chemotherapeutic agents that act as local vesicants. Drugs particularly likely to cause necrosis upon extravasation include doxorubicin, actinomycin D, mitomycin C, and vincristine. Because antidotes are largely ineffective, preventing extravasation injury is the key. As a result, these drugs should only be administered via a freely flowing intravenous line with careful monitoring.

Other toxicities are possible with chemotherapeutic agents administered alone or in combination. The package insert that accompanies all commercially available anticancer agents details the specific toxicities associated with each agent and should be reviewed before the administration of unfamiliar agents.

■■■ Dose Adjustments for Chemotherapeutic Toxicity

Different patients respond differently to chemotherapeutic regimens, and it is important to modify treatment doses in accordance with each patient's individual tolerance. A variety of modification programs have been developed, and one of the most useful sources of these dose-modification programs are the clinical protocols developed by the National Cooperative Groups. One example of a typical dose modification program is the so-called sliding scale of drug-dose adjusting for the degree of myelosuppression seen with prior doses of chemotherapy. Doses of myelosuppressive chemotherapeutic agents are reduced if the patient experiences significant bone marrow suppression or the recovery time from that bone marrow suppression is substantially prolonged. Dose-limiting toxicities in other organ systems require alternative sliding scales based on other drug-related toxicities.

Selected Reading

Bookman MA, Young RC: Principles of chemotherapy in gynecologic cancer, Chapter 15. In WJ Hoskins, CA Perez, and RC Young (eds.), *Principles and Practice of Gynecologic Oncology*. Lippincott Williams & Williams, Philadelphia, 2000, pp. 403–424.

Calvert AH, Newell LA, Grumbell LA, et al: Carboplatin dosage: Prospective evaluation of a simple formula based on renal function. *J Clin Oncol* 1989; 7:1748.

Chu E, DeVita VT: Principles of cancer management: chemotherapy, Chapter 17. In VT DeVita, S Hellman, SA Rosenberg (eds.), *Cancer: Principles and Practice of Oncology*. Lippincott Williams & Williams, Philadelphia, 2001, pp. 289–306.

Kaufman DC, Chabner BA: Clinical strategies for cancer treatment: the role of drugs, Chapter 1. In BA Chabner, Longo DL (eds.), *Cancer Chemotherapy and Biotherapy: Principles and Practice*. Lippincott Williams & Williams, Philadelphia, 2001, pp. 1–16.

Levin L, Hyrniuk W: Dose intensity analysis of chemotherapy regimens in ovarian cancer. *J Clin Oncol* 1987; 5:756.

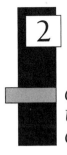

2

CHEMOTHERAPEUTIC AGENTS USED IN THE TREATMENT OF GYNECOLOGIC MALIGNANCIES

JAKOB DUPONT, MIKA A. SOVAK, IVOR BENJAMIN, AND DAVID SPRIGGS

Modern chemotherapeutic regimens for the treatment of gynecologic malignancies utilize a wide variety of agents with different chemical properties and mechanisms of action. An understanding of the chemistry, mechanism of action, clinical pharmacology, pharmacokinetics, dosage schedule, and toxicity profile of the various agents, used alone or in combination, is essential for the practicing gynecologic oncologist.

This chapter focuses on the frequently used agents for gynecologic malignancies. Particular emphasis will be placed on developing rationale for appropriate usage of these agents. Justification for multidrug combinations, route of administration, or duration of administration is often best understood in the context of the mechanism of action of the individual agents.

Chemotherapeutic agents are often classified either by their chemical origin or by the phase of the cell cycle when they are active. In terms of chemical derivation, remarkably diverse compounds share activity against gynecologic malignancies. These include antimetabolites, alkylating agents, antitumor antibiotics, plant alkaloids, taxanes, hormonal agents, monoclonal antibodies, and targeted therapies (Table 2.1). Several general reference texts are included in Selected Reading at the end of the chapter.

Chemotherapy of Gynecologic Cancers: Society of Gynecologic Oncologists Handbook 2e, edited by Stephen C. Rubin, MD, Lippincott Williams & Wilkins, Philadelphia © 2004.

Table 2.1

Classification of Commonly Used Chemotherapeutic Agents for Gynecologic Malignancies

Class	Drug	Common Application in Gynecologic Oncology
Antimetabolites	Methotrexate	GTD
	Fluorouracil	Cervix
	Capecitabine	EOC, cervix
	Gemcitabine	EOC, sarc
Alkylating agents	Cyclophosphamide	EOC, GTD
	Ifosfamide	Cervix, EOC, sarc
	Melphalan	Cervix, EOC
	Cisplatin	Cervix, endometrial, EOC, GC, GTD, vagina, vulva
	Carboplatin	Cervix, endometrial, ECC, GC, GTD, vagina, vulva
	Oxaliplatin	EOC
	Chlorambucil	EOC, GTD
	Altretamine	EOC
Antitumor antibiotics	Dactinomycin	GTD
	Bleomycin	GC, vulva
	Doxorubicin	EOC, cervix, endometrial, breast, vulva
	Liposomal doxorubicin	EOC
	Mitomycin C	Cervix
	Mitoxantrone	EOC
Agents derived from plants	Vinblastine	Breast, GC, GTD
	Vincristine	Breast, GC, GTD
	Vinorelbine	EOC, cervix
	Etoposide	EOC, GTD, GC, Sarc
	Paclitaxel	EOC, breast, endometrial
	Docetaxel	EOC
	Topotecan	EOC
	Irinotecan	EOC

(continues)

█████ Table 2.1 (cont'd.)

Class	Drug	Common Application in Gynecologic Oncology
Hormonal agents	Megestrol acetate	Endometrial, breast, ESS
	Tamoxifen citrate	Breast, EOC
Monoclonal antibodies	Ovarex	EOC
	Cetuximab	EOC
Targeted therapy	Iressa	EOC
	OSI-774	EOC
	Bortezomib	EOC

Breast, breast carcinoma; cervix, cervical carcinoma; endometrial, endometrial carcinoma; EOC, epithelial ovarian carcinoma; ESS, endometrial stromal sarcoma; GC, ovarian germ cell tumor; GTD, gestational trophoblastic disease; sarc, ovarian and uterine sarcomas; vagina, vaginal carcinoma; vulva, vulvar carcinoma.

█████ *Antimetabolites*

The antimetabolites are structural and chemical analogs of naturally occurring substances in the metabolic pathways leading to the synthesis of purines, pyrimidines, and nucleic acids. In most cases, they are S phase–specific agents that are most effective in rapidly growing tumors associated with short doubling times and large growth fractions. Because of the cycle-specific mechanism of action, efficacy of antimetabolites is dependent on duration of exposure. Therefore, long exposure is often more effective. The antimetabolites may be subclassified into purine analogs (6-mercaptopurine), fluorinated pyrimidines (fluorouracil), ribonucleotide reductase inhibitors (hydroxyurea), and folic acid antagonists (methotrexate). The toxicity profile of antimetabolites usually reflects damage to rapidly dividing normal tissues. Therefore, stomatitis, diarrhea, and myelosuppression are typically seen. The carcinogenic potential of the antimetabolites is thought to be low and secondary malignancies are rare.

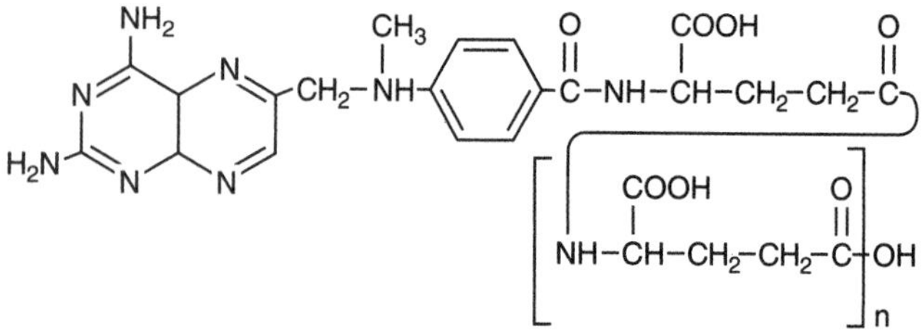

Figure 2.1.
Chemical structure of methotrexate. Reproduced with permission from Perry MC: *The Chemotherapy Source Book*, 1st edition. Williams & Wilkins, Baltimore, 1992, p. 1172.

■■■■ Methotrexate

CHEMISTRY

Methotrexate (MTX) is a 4-amino, 10-methyl analog of aminopterin. Its chemical structure is shown in Fig. 2.1.

MECHANISM OF ACTION

The classic model for the antitumor activity of MTX is the inhibition of dihydrofolate reductase that leads to depletion of the intracellular reduced tetrahydrofolate pool. Inhibition of dihydrofolate reductase will result in depletion of reduced folate and thymidine starvation. However, cell line studies imply that mechanisms other than thymidine depletion contribute to the cytotoxicity of methotrexate. Cancer cells exposed to prolonged high concentrations of MTX lead to an incomplete depletion of intracellular reduced folates, yet DNA synthesis was decreased to less than 20% of controls. MTX also inhibits the *de novo* synthesis of purine nucleosides, and consequently inhibits both DNA and RNA synthesis.

CLINICAL PHARMACOLOGY AND PHARMACOKINETICS

Drug concentration and duration of exposure are the two most important contributors to MTX cytotoxicity. There appears to be a specific, tissue-dependent threshold for inhibition of DNA synthesis induced by methotrexate. After an intravenous injection, MTX distributes in a volume approximately equal to that of total body water. At higher doses, bioavailability becomes erratic as the carrier-mediated transport mechanism in the bowel becomes saturated. Approximately 60% of the drug is bound to serum albumin. In general, MTX exhibits three phases of clearance from the serum. Most of the MTX in the serum undergoes renal excretion, though a small fraction is eliminated in the bile. MTX undergoes glomerular filtration in addition to active secretion by the proximal renal tubules. The first phase, lasting 40 to 50 minutes, is an initial distribution phase. This is followed by the second phase, lasting 12 to 24 hours, during which the half-life is 2 or 3 hours. During the terminal phase of clearance, the half-life increases to 8 to 10 hours. Because methotrexate toxicity correlates with duration of exposure, renal impairment may greatly increase toxicity. Therefore, adequate renal function should be documented before therapy is initiated. This evaluation would include a normal serum creatinine and creatinine clearance of at least 60 mL/min.

MTX readily distributes into ascitic or pleural fluid collections, binding to proteins. This may significantly alter the pharmacokinetics by increasing the terminal half-life. Patients with third-space fluid collections are at very high risk for methotrexate toxicity.

DOSAGE AND SCHEDULES

When given as part of the EMA-CO regimen (etoposide-methotrexate-dactinomycin and cyclophosphamide-vincristine) for high-risk gestational trophoblastic disease:

> *Day 1:* 100 mg/m^2 i.v. bolus is followed by 200 mg/m^2 as a 12-hour i.v. infusion
> *Day 2:* 15 mg folinic acid i.m. or PO q6h × 4 doses; begin 12 hours after MTX infusion is completed
> (repeat every 14 days)

In cases with CNS metastases, the day 1 MTX dose is increased to 1,000 mg/m^2 as a 24-hour i.v. infusion. In addition, 12.5 mg of MTX is given via intrathecal injection. On day 2, the folinic acid dose is increased to 15 mg q8h × 9 doses. If renal insufficiency or injury is present, high-dose MTX is a dangerous regimen that requires prospective MTX concentration monitoring and concentration-directed folinic acid rescue.

When given as a single agent for nonmetastatic or low-risk metastatic gestational trophoblastic disease:

Regimen 1: 15 to 30 mg MTX i.m. daily for 5 days (repeat every 7 days)
Regimen 2: 1 mg/kg MTX i.m. on days 1, 3, 5, and 7
13 mg folinic acid p.o. 30 hours after each methotrexate dose

TOXICITY

HEMATOLOGIC

Myelosuppression: 5 to 14 days after administration

DERMATOLOGIC

Alopecia

GASTROINTESTINAL

Mucositis: 3 to 7 days after administration

HEPATIC

Elevation of liver enzymes and bilirubin within 10 days after administration

RENAL

Nephrotoxicity results from precipitation of MTX and metabolites in renal tubules. Avoid by vigorous hydration and urinary alkalization. When renal function is impaired, monitoring of serum methotrexate levels is advised in order to guide dosage and duration of folinic acid administration.

PULMONARY

Pneumonitis: usually self-limiting

NEUROLOGIC

Meningitis: associated with intrathecal therapy

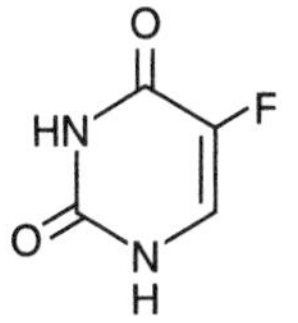

Figure 2.2.
Chemical structure of 5-FU. Reproduced with permission from Perry MC: *The Chemotherapy Source Book*, 1st edition. Williams & Wilkins, Baltimore, 1992, p. 1172.

Fluorouracil

CHEMISTRY

Fluorouracil (5-FU) is a fluoropyrimidine with the chemical name 5-fluoro2,4(1H,3H) pyrimidinedione. It is sensitive to light and may precipitate at room temperature. The chemical structure of 5-FU is shown in Fig. 2.2.

MECHANISM OF ACTION

In 1957, Heidelberger synthesized 5-FU with the intention of developing a novel cytotoxic agent. The theoretical basis for this development stemmed from the observation that tumor cells utilized uracil more efficiently than normal cells of the intestinal mucosa. 5-FU is inactive until it is converted into one of its many cytotoxic metabolites by the target tissue. Although the exact mechanism of action of 5-FU remains to be determined, it appears that the inhibition of thymidylate synthase by the active metabolite 5-FdUMP and reduced folates leads to the formation of an inactive ternary complex. This may be enhanced by coadministration of folinic acid. Inhibition of thymidylate synthase leads to inhibition of DNA synthesis through the depletion of thymidine pools. Sequence-dependent interaction between 5-FU and MTX is well established. MTX and 5-FU are maximally synergistic when the MTX is given 24 hours before 5-FU, inhibiting the production of normal purine precursors. As an alternative mechanism of action, FUTP incorporation into RNA and subsequent impaired RNA function may have a role. 5-FdUTP incorporation into DNA as a fraudulent thymidine precursor may induce single-strand breaks and produce cytotoxic effects.

CLINICAL PHARMACOLOGY AND PHARMACOKINETICS

5-FU is usually given intravenously. Bioavailability after oral administration is highly variable because of an inconsistent absorption from the gastrointestinal tract and first-pass metabolism to inactive compounds by the liver. A typical intravenous injection of 10 to 15 mg/kg results in peak plasma concentrations of 0.1 to 1.0 mM. It is uncertain if 5-FU is cleared via two or three phases of elimination. Less than 10% of 5-FU is bound to serum proteins. CSF levels are less than 2% of plasma levels. The half-life is short (6–20 minutes), owing to rapid metabolism by the liver and other tissues. Over 80% of 5-FU is metabolized to dihydrofluorouracil, which is further metabolized and excreted in the urine. Approximately 15% of administered 5-FU is excreted unchanged in the urine. The hepatic detoxification of 5-FU allows for high-dose portal vein administration for the treatment of liver metastases with minimal systemic toxicity.

DOSAGE AND SCHEDULES

When given for the treatment of recurrent cervical cancer:

Usual dosage: 5-FU 750 to 1000 mg/m^2/day over a 4- or 5-day continuous i.v. infusion

This course is usually repeated in 28-day intervals

TOXICITY

HEMATOLOGIC
Myelosuppression: 9 to 14 days after administration

GASTROINTESTINAL
Diarrhea: watery, may be life threatening
Stomatitis
Hepatic: associated with portal administration
Mucositis: 3 to 7 days after administration
Hepatotoxicity: elevation of liver enzymes and bilirubin within 10 days after administration

DERMATOLOGIC
Dermatitis

Photosensitivity
Hyperpigmentation
Nail changes

NEUROLOGIC

Cerebellar syndrome (headache, ataxia, nystagmus, confusion)
Cerebellar injury is usually reversible but may be permanent

CARDIAC

Ischemia, angina, and infarction (rare)

OCULAR

Keratitis leading to lacrimal duct stenosis and increased lacrimation in addition to blurred vision and photophobia
Nasal discharge

Capecitabine (Xeloda)

CHEMISTRY

Capecitabine is an oral prodrug of 5-FU. The chemical structure of capecitabine is shown in Fig. 2.3.

MECHANISM OF ACTION

Capecitabine is an oral prodrug that is ultimately converted in tumor tissue to the active cytotoxic agent 5-FU. The mechanism of action of capecitabine is the same as that of 5-FU, within cancer cells.

CLINICAL PHARMACOLOGY AND PHARMACOKINETICS

Capecitabine is an oral chemotherapeutic agent. It is eliminated in the urine and the elimination half-life is about 45 minutes. Food reduces the rate and extent of absorption of capecitabine. Capecitabine should be taken in divided doses, 12 hours apart. It should be administered, with water, 30 minutes after a meal. The pharmacokinetics of capecitabine and its metabolites are dose-dependent over a dosage range of 500 to 3,500 mg/m^2/day.

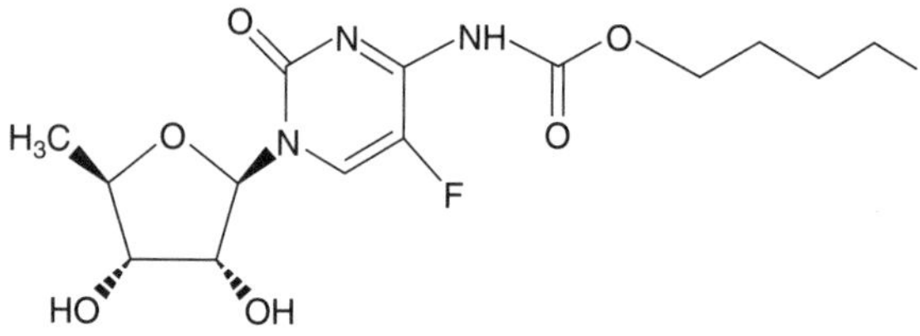

Capecitabine

Figure 2.3.
Chemical structure of capecitabine.

DOSAGE AND SCHEDULE

When given for recurrent cervical or epithelial ovarian cancer:

Standard dosing is 1,500 to 2,000 mg/m^2 daily in two divided doses for 2 weeks with a 1-week rest period (repeat every 3 weeks). Capecitabine dosing is modified in the presence of mild to moderate renal insufficiency (creatinine clearance 30–50 mL/minute). Patients with severe renal insufficiency (creatinine clearance less than 30) should not receive capecitabine.

TOXICITY

HEMATOLOGIC

Myelosuppression

GASTROINTESTINAL

Diarrhea
Vomiting
Nausea
Stomatitis
Abdominal pain
Constipation
Dyspepsia

DERMATOLOGIC

Hand and foot syndrome (palmar-plantar erythrodysesthesia syndrome) characterized by painful erythema and
edema

HEPATIC

Hyperbilirubinemia

■■■ Gemcitabine (Gemzar)

CHEMISTRY

Gemcitabine is a deoxycytidine analog with the chemical
name 2,2-difluorodeoxycytidine. The chemical structure is
shown in Fig. 2.4.

MECHANISM OF ACTION

Gemcitabine is actively transported into cells where phos-
phorylation converts the parent compound into gemcitabine triphosphate, the active metabolite. Cytotoxicity is
mediated through several mechanisms. The direct inhibition of ribonucleotide reductase blocks the conversion of ri-
bonucleotides to deoxyribonucleotides, thus blocking DNA

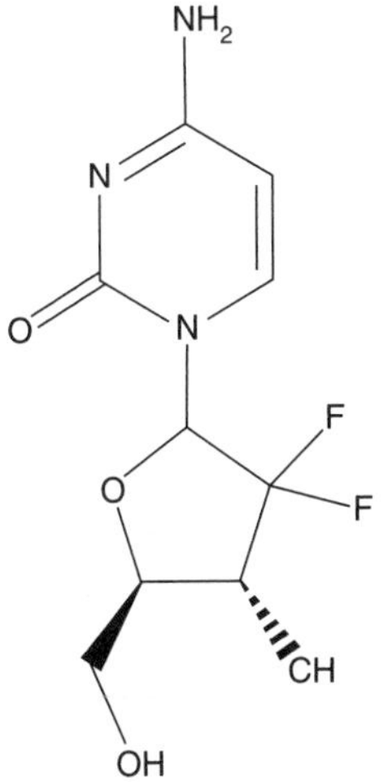

Figure 2.4.
Chemical structure of gemcitabine.

synthesis. The active drug is also incorporated into DNA, resulting in strand termination. In addition, there is inhibition of DNA polymerase. Notable is the fact that the activity of gemcitabine is not limited to the S phase of cell growth, suggesting that there may be other unknown mechanisms of action.

CLINICAL PHARMACOLOGY AND PHARMACOKINETICS

Gemcitabine is minimally protein bound, and has a high volume of distribution. Peak plasma concentrations are found within 30 minutes of drug administration. The half-life of the parent compound is approximately 1 hour, though the active metabolite can be detected in the plasma for up to 24 hours after administration. Clearance is predominantly renal. A fixed dose rate infusion of 10 mg/m^2/minute has been more effective than 30-minute infusion in pancreatic cancer, but has more myelosuppression as well.

DOSAGE AND SCHEDULES

When given to patients with epithelial ovarian cancer:

Days 1, 8, 15: 800 to 1,000 mg/m^2 i.v.; repeat every 28 days
Days 1, 8: 800 to 1,000 mg/m^2 i.v.; repeat every 21 days

When given to patients with leiomyosarcoma:

Days 1, 8: 900 mg/m^2 i.v.; repeat every 21 days

TOXICITY

HEMATOLOGIC
Myelosuppression, particularly thrombocytopenia

GASTROINTESTINAL
Nausea
Vomiting
Change in bowel habits
Stomatitis

DERMATOLOGIC
Radiation recall
Maculopapular rash

HEPATIC
Transaminitis
Elevation in bilirubin and alkaline phosphatase

RENAL
Hemolytic-uremic syndrome
Hematuria
Proteinuria

PULMONARY
Acute respiratory distress syndrome

NEUROLOGIC
Somnolence
Headache

HYPERSENSITIVITY
Acute infusion-associated reaction, characterized by dyspnea, flushing, chills, headache, back pain, and hypotension, can occur in up to 5% of patients.

OTHER
Flu-like symptoms (common)
Asthenia (common)
Peripheral edema

▬ *Alkylating Agents*

The alkylating agents are a diverse array of chemical compounds. They were among the first agents applied to the treatment of cancer. They are highly reactive substances that share common chemical properties. They all possess positively charged alkyl groups that are able to bind to negatively charged (electron-rich) sites on DNA.

The cytotoxicity of the alkylating agents comes from their ability to form DNA adducts, leading to single- or double-stranded breaks or cross-links. DNA alkylation most commonly occurs at the N-7 position of guanine. Adducts also occur at a lower frequency at the N-1 and O-6 positions of guanine, N-1, N-3, and N-7 positions of adenine, N-3 position of cytosine, and O-4 position of thymidine.

In addition to the direct effects of alkylating agents by the formation of adducts, repair mechanisms may be unsuccessful in attempting to restore the integrity of DNA, leading to further damage. Therefore, agents that inhibit enzymes in the DNA repair process may be used as modulators to increase the cytotoxicity of alkylating agents. The fact that repair mechanisms are saturable provides a rationale for high-dose alkylating agent therapy.

The sulfhydryl groups on intracellular glutathione and metallothionein provide an alternative target for the alkylating agents and thereby confer resistance to these drugs. Overexpression of the protein metallothionein contributes to resistance. Buthionine sulfoximine has been shown to positively modulate the effects of various alkylating agents by inhibiting the rate-limiting enzyme (γ-glutamyl cysteine synthetase) in the biosynthetic pathway to glutathione, reducing intracellular glutathione levels.

Although alkylating agents share a common mechanism of action, they differ greatly in their clinical pharmacokinetic toxicity profiles. The platinum analogs, also discussed in this section, are not true alkylating agents. Rather, they form adducts between DNA and their platinum atom. The end result, however, is an analogous covalent bond to DNA with distortion of the double helix.

■■■ Cyclophosphamide

CHEMISTRY

Cyclophosphamide is an alkylating agent with the chemical name 2-[bis(2-chloroethyl)-amino]tetrahydro-2H-1,3,2-oxazaphosphorine 2-oxide monohydrate. The chemical structure is shown in Fig. 2.5.

MECHANISM OF ACTION

As with most alkylating agents, the cytotoxic effects of cyclophosphamide are mediated via the formation of DNA adducts, which distort the secondary and tertiary structures of DNA. Cyclophosphamide is notable for requiring a mul-

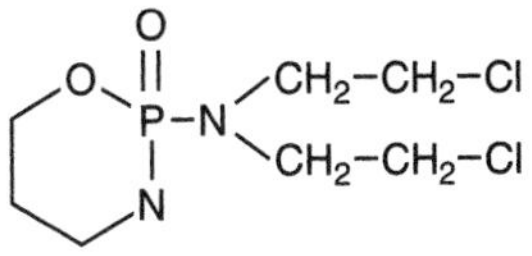

Figure 2.5.
Chemical structure of
cyclophosphamide.

tistep metabolic activation to confer antitumor activity. This activation occurs via the hepatic P-450 microsomal enzyme system and results in the formation of the active alkylating agent 4-OH-cyclophosphamide. This compound further degenerates to other active compounds (aldophosphamide and phosphoramide mustard) and inactive compounds (acrolein, nornitrogen mustard, carboxyphosphamide, and 4-ketocyclophosphamide). This metabolic pathway is illustrated in Fig. 2.6.

CLINICAL PHARMACOLOGY AND PHARMACOKINETICS

Cyclophosphamide is readily absorbed after oral administration with a bioavailability of over 90%. It reaches a peak plasma concentration at approximately 1 hour. However, the drug is usually given intravenously. Approximately 12% of cyclophosphamide is excreted unchanged in the urine. The remainder is metabolized via liver enzymes into multiple active metabolites that are then excreted in the urine. Cyclophosphamide has a half-life of elimination of 3–10 hours.

DOSAGE AND SCHEDULES

When given as part of a combination regimen for epithelial ovarian carcinoma:

> *Cyclophosphamide:* 750 to 1,000 mg/m^2 i.v. in 100–250 cc normal saline over at least 15 minutes, with hydration

When given as part of a regimen for epithelial ovarian cancer that includes peripheral stem-cell harvesting:

> *Cyclophosphamide:* 3 to 6 g/m^2 i.v. in divided doses within a 24-hour period

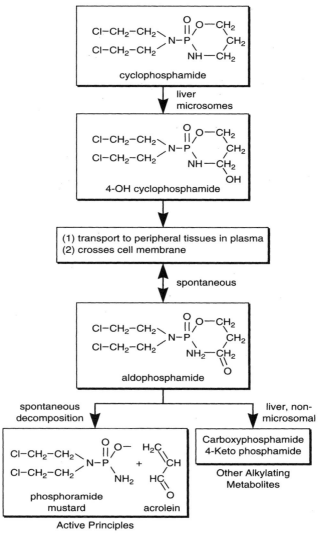

Figure 2.6.
Metabolism of cyclophosphamide.

Mesna (N-acetylcysteine, sodium, 2-mercaptoethane sulfonate) as a bladder protectant may be given as a continuous i.v. infusion of up to 4.5 g/m^2/day during high-dose cyclophosphamide therapy

When given as part of the EMA-CO regimen (etoposide-methotrexate-dactinomycin and cyclophosphamide-vincristine) for high-risk gestational trophoblastic disease:

Cyclophosphamide: 600 mg/m^2 i.v.; repeat every 14 days.

TOXICITY

HEMATOLOGIC

Myelosuppression: 8 to 14 days after administration: tends to be brief in duration and cumulative toxicity is uncommon
Secondary leukemias

GASTROINTESTINAL

Nausea/vomiting: often delayed 6–8 hours after administration
Antiemetic prophylaxis is recommended for 24 hours

DERMATOLOGIC

Alopecia (common)
Skin pigmentation
Nail changes
Dermatitis
Facial flushing

HEPATIC

Increased serum glutamic oxaloacetic transaminase (SGOT)/serum glutamate pyruvate transaminase (SGPT) (uncommon), hepatitis/jaundice (rare)

GENITOURINARY

Hemorrhagic cystitis (common with high-dose therapy)
Bladder fibrosis (rare)

NEUROLOGIC

Headaches
Dizziness
Metallic taste during injection

CARDIAC

Cardiac necrosis (rare with high-dose therapy)

Myopericarditis (rare with high-dose therapy)

PULMONARY

Interstitial fibrosis (rare)

■■■ Ifosfamide

CHEMISTRY

Ifosfamide is an alkylating agent with the chemical name 1,3,2oxazaphosphorine,3-(2-chloroethyl)-2-[(2-chlorethyl)-amino]tetrahydro-2-oxide. It has a similar oxazaphosphorine ring structure as cyclophosphamide. The chemical structure of ifosfamide is shown in Fig. 2.7.

MECHANISM OF ACTION

The mechanism of action of ifosfamide is typical for the alkylating agents. It appears to be mediated by the formation of DNA adducts. Ifosfamide, like cyclophosphamide, is notable for requiring activation via the hepatic microsomal enzyme system. Ifosfamide is activated more slowly than cyclophosphamide and forms proportionally less active alkylating agent (ifosfamide mustard). Therefore, larger doses are required for equivalent efficacy since more is excreted in the urine when compared with cyclophosphamide.

CLINICAL PHARMACOLOGY AND PHARMACOKINETICS

Ifosfamide is readily absorbed after oral administration with a bioavailability of 100%. Dose-dependent pharmacokinetics are observed. In the 3.8- to 5.0-g/m^2 dose range, elimination is biphasic with a half-life of 16 hours. At lower doses, elimination is linear with a half-life of 6.9 hours. At

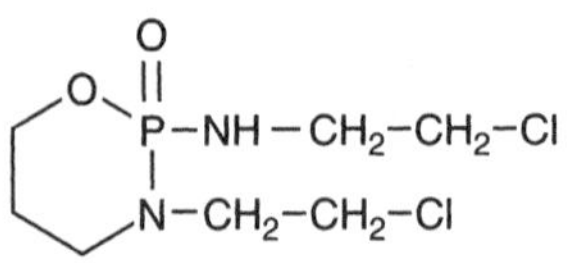

Figure 2.7.
Chemical structure of ifosfamide.

higher doses, up to 60% of the drug is excreted inactivated in the urine. Activation is more efficient at lower doses (less than 2.4 g/m^2) with less than 20% of the infused dose excreted unaltered, implying that the hepatic microsomal activation of ifosfamide is saturable. This provides a rationale for multiday continuous infusions. Patients with renal insufficiency are at higher risk for ifosfamide toxicity.

DOSAGE AND SCHEDULES

When given as part of a combination regimen for epithelial ovarian carcinoma or recurrent cervical carcinoma:

Ifosfamide: 1.0 to 2.5 g/m^2/day i.v. over 2 to 5 days; repeat every 21 days

Mesna (N-acetylcysteine, sodium, 2-mercaptoethane sulfonate) as a bladder protectant: 400 mg/m^2 i.v. at 15 minutes, 4 hours, and 8 hours after ifosfamide infusion; may be given orally at 800 mg/m^2; alternatively, it should be given as a continuous infusion when ifosfamide is given continuously

TOXICITY

HEMATOLOGIC

Myelosuppression: 7 to 10 days after administration
Secondary leukemias

GASTROINTESTINAL

Nausea/vomiting: antiemetic prophylaxis is recommended

DERMATOLOGIC

Alopecia (common)
Skin pigmentation
Nail changes
Dermatitis
Facial flushing

HEPATIC

Increased SGOT/SGPT (uncommon)

GENITOURINARY

Hemorrhagic cystitis (common when mesna is not used)
Bladder fibrosis (rare)

NEUROLOGIC

Syndrome with any combination of somnolence, lethargy, ataxia, confusion, disorientation, dizziness, malaise, and in severe cases, coma.

These toxicities are more commonly associated with:

1-day versus 5-day regimen
Renal insufficiency
Hypoalbuminemia
Concomitant sedative usage

Melphalan (Alkeran)

CHEMISTRY

Melphalan is an alkylating agent that is a phenylalanine derivative of nitrogen mustard. It has the chemical name 4-[bis(2-chloroethyl)-amino]-L-phenylalanine. The chemical structure of melphalan is shown in Fig. 2.8.

MECHANISM OF ACTION

The mechanism of action of melphalan is typical for the alkylating agents. Its action is dependent on the formation of DNA adducts. Being a phenylalanine derivative, melphalan is actively transported into cells via the L-amino acid transport system. Several drugs are known to impair the uptake, and therefore efficacy, of melphalan. These include doxorubicin, aminophylline, chlorpromazine, indomethacin, and tamoxifen.

CLINICAL PHARMACOLOGY AND PHARMACOKINETICS

Melphalan is inconsistently absorbed after oral administration with a bioavailability of 25% to 90%. Peak plasma con-

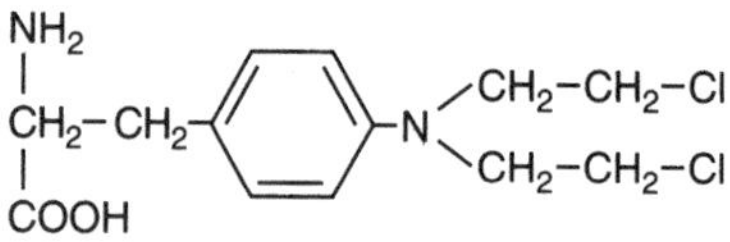

Figure 2.8.
Chemical structure of melphalan.

centrations are reached 2 hours after an oral dose. Over 80% of circulating melphalan is bound to plasma proteins. The drug has a half-life of elimination of 1.5 to 4 hours.

DOSAGE AND SCHEDULES

When given as part of a combination regimen for epithelial ovarian carcinoma or recurrent cervical carcinoma:

> *Melphalan:* 0.2 mg/kg i.v. daily for 5 days, repeated every 4 weeks

TOXICITY

HEMATOLOGIC

Myelosuppression: leukopenia and thrombocytopenia with prolonged recovery (6–8 weeks)
Secondary malignancies

GASTROINTESTINAL

Nausea/vomiting
Mucositis
Diarrhea

DERMATOLOGIC

Dermatitis
Pruritus
Rash
Alopecia (common)

HYPERSENSITIVITY

Urticaria (rare)
Anaphylaxis (rare)

■ Cisplatin

CHEMISTRY

Cisplatin is an organoplatinum complex with the chemical name *cis*-diamminedichloroplatinum (II). The oxidation state of the platinum atom is $+2$. Its antitumor activity is highly dependent on the stereospecificity of the *cis* configuration. The chemical structures of cisplatin and the closely related drugs carboplatin and oxaliplatin are shown in Fig. 2.9.

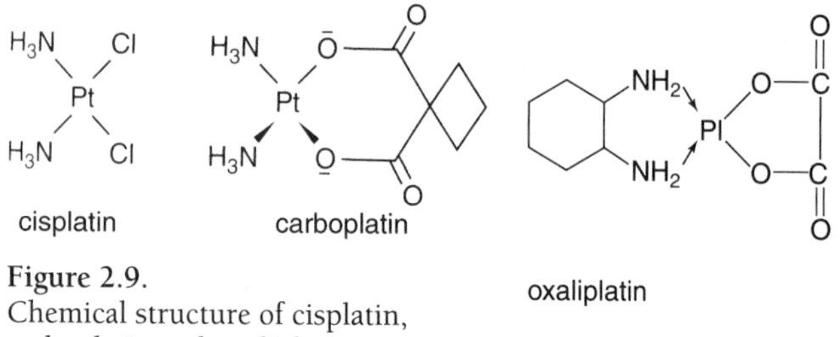

Figure 2.9.
Chemical structure of cisplatin, carboplatin and oxaliplatin.

MECHANISM OF ACTION

The mechanism of action of cisplatin is similar to that of the true alkylating agents. Antitumor activity is mediated via the formation of platinum adducts with DNA. Cisplatin differs from the true alkylating agents in that the covalent bonds with DNA are formed with the platinum atom. These heavy-metal adducts distort the DNA double helix by bending it up to 40 degrees and thereby maintaining the planar stereochemistry diamineplatinum (II) complex. The presence of the platinum adducts and the bending of the double helix probably are the major contributors to inhibition of DNA synthesis. However, the precise mechanism by which DNA adducts lead to cell death remains to be determined.

After intravenous administration, cisplatin exists in the bloodstream in its native dichloro form. Circulating cisplatin remains in the dichloro form because of the relatively high chloride concentration in the plasma (approximately 100 mmol). This dichloro form enters cells in the target tissues via passive diffusion. The drug must undergo aquation hydrolysis, leading to the active diaquo form. This is facilitated by the low intracellular chloride concentration of approximately 4 mmol.

The highly reactive diaquo species binds preferentially to the N7 positions of guanine and adenine. Additionally, cisplatin binds to other macromolecules including RNA and proteins. On a molar basis, cisplatin is more reactive with RNA than DNA. However, the cytotoxic effects of cisplatin in cell culture are highly correlated with platinum-DNA adduct formation.

Two common platinum-DNA adducts account for over 90% of the adducts observed. An N7-diammineplatinum-d adduct involving two adjacent guanine bases on the same DNA strand is referred to as d(GpG). This is the most commonly formed adduct, accounting for roughly 60% of all platinum-DNA interactions. The analogous d(ApG) adduct where platinum is bound to the N7 of adenine and an adjacent guanine on the same DNA strand accounts for approximately 30% of observed adducts. The remaining 10% of adducts are a mixture of d(Gp × pG), interstrand cross-linking adducts, and monoadducts. The four most common cisplatin-DNA adducts are shown in Fig. 2.10.

CLINICAL PHARMACOLOGY AND PHARMACOKINETICS

Following intravenous administration, cisplatin is rapidly and extensively protein bound. Over 90% is bound to plasma proteins within 4 hours of administration. Clearance of cisplatin is triphasic. The first two phases of elimination, lasting 20 to 30 minutes and 50 to 70 minutes respectively, represent removal of drug that is not bound to plasma pro-

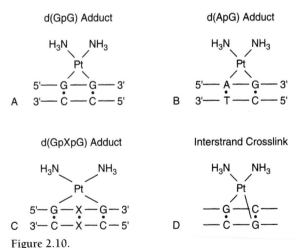

Figure 2.10.
Common cisplatin-DNA adducts.

teins. The third phase, lasting approximately 24 hours, represents elimination of inactivated cisplatin bound to circulating proteins. Over 90% of the elimination is via a combination of glomerular filtration and tubular secretion. After intraperitoneal administration, a local pharmacologic advantage of 21 times plasma concentrations is attainable. Over 50% of cisplatin instilled into the peritoneal cavity is absorbed into the systemic circulation.

DOSAGE AND SCHEDULES

The following pertain to cisplatin given as part of a combination regimen for a variety of gynecologic malignancies:

Intravenous: 50 to 100 mg/m^2 over 30 minutes with vigorous hydration before and after therapy; repeated every 3 weeks

Intraperitoneal: 50 to 100 mg/m^2 in 2 L over 30 minutes with vigorous hydration before and after therapy; repeated every 3 weeks

TOXICITY

HEMATOLOGIC

Myelosuppression: all three cell lineages are affected, although the anemia is primarily mediated through renal toxicity

GASTROINTESTINAL

Nausea/vomiting (common, severe); aggressive antiemetic prophylaxis with serotonin antagonists is recommended
Diarrhea (rare)

DERMATOLOGIC

Alopecia (uncommon)
Discoloration of the nails

HEPATIC

Increased SGOT/SGPT (rare)

NEUROLOGIC

Peripheral neuropathy (common and often dose limiting)
Numbness and tingling

Ototoxicity (high-frequency loss and tinnitus)
Autonomic neuropathy (dizziness)
Other neurologic toxicities (uncommon)
Agitation
Paranoia
Cortical blindness
Seizures
Fatigue
Raynaud's phenomenon (rare)

RENAL

Nephrotoxicity, both glomerular and tubular injury (common and cumulative)
Hypomagnesemia (common)
Hypokalemia (common)

CARDIOVASCULAR

Bradycardia (rare)
Congestive heart failure (rare)

■■■ Carboplatin

CHEMISTRY

Carboplatin is a platinum-containing alkylating-like agent with the chemical name *cis*-diammine [1,1-cyclobutane dicarboxylato'(2-)0,0'] platinum (II). The oxidation state of the platinum atom is +2. Its antitumor activity is highly dependent on the stereospecificity of the *cis* configuration. The chemical structure is shown in Fig. 2.9.

MECHANISM OF ACTION

Carboplatin was the first cisplatin analog to be approved for clinical use. The mechanism of action of carboplatin is similar to that of cisplatin. Antitumor activity is mediated via the formation of platinum adducts with DNA. Carboplatin differs from the true alkylating agents in that the covalent bonds with DNA are formed with the platinum atom. These heavy-metal adducts distort the DNA double helix by bending it up to 40 degrees and thereby maintaining the planar stereochemistry diammineplatinum (II) complex. The presence of the platinum adducts and the bending of the double helix probably are the major contributors to inhibition of DNA synthesis. However, the precise mechanism by which DNA adducts lead to cell death remains to be determined.

Carboplatin also undergoes a similar, albeit slower, aquation reaction like cisplatin, leading to the active diaquo species. The highly reactive diaquo species binds preferentially to the N7 positions of guanine and adenine. Refer to the section on cisplatin earlier in this chapter for a discussion of specific adducts.

CLINICAL PHARMACOLOGY AND PHARMACOKINETICS

After intravenous administration, carboplatin is rapidly cleared from the serum via glomerular filtration. Triphasic elimination is observed. The initial phase lasts only 15 to 30 minutes, the second phase lasts 80 to 100 minutes, and the terminal phase is 22 to 40 hours. The lack of tubular excretion probably contributes to carboplatin's lower nephrotoxicity when compared with cisplatin. However, being that the elimination of carboplatin is highly dependent on the glomerular filtration rate, dose adjustment is indicated in the setting of renal failure in order to minimize myelotoxicity.

DOSAGE AND SCHEDULES

When given as part of a combination regimen for a variety of gynecologic malignancies:

Carboplatin: 360 to 400 mg/m^2 i.v. over 30 minutes; repeat every 21–28 days

Much higher doses have been used in various dose-intensification protocols with stem cell or bone marrow transplantation support. Most authorities recommend pharmacokinetically guided dosing to area under the curve (AUC) values of 5.0 to 8.0. The dose (in mg/m^2) may be calculated using the formula described by Calvert (1989):

Dose (mg) = target AUC × (creatinine clearance + 25)

TOXICITY

HEMATOLOGIC

Myelosuppression: thrombocytopenia (at 14–21 days after administration) is much more severe than with cisplatin and is dose limiting

GASTROINTESTINAL

Nausea/vomiting (less severe than cisplatin); antiemetic prophylaxis is recommended

Diarrhea

DERMATOLOGIC

Alopecia (uncommon)

HEPATIC

Increased SGOT/SGPT (uncommon)

NEUROLOGIC

Peripheral neuropathy (rare when compared with cisplatin)

RENAL

Nephrotoxicity (uncommon when compared with cisplatin)

Hypomagnesemia (uncommon when compared with cisplatin)

▰ Oxaliplatin

CHEMISTRY

Oxaliplatin is a cisplatin analog. It is the first available diaminocyclohexane platinum derivative. The chemical structure is shown in Fig. 2.9.

MECHANISM OF ACTION

The mechanism of action of oxaliplatin is thought to be similar to that of cisplatin. Cisplatin cross-resistance is less likely with oxaliplatin than with carboplatin because oxaliplatin adducts are not substrates for the mismatch repair system.

CLINICAL PHARMACOLOGY AND PHARMACOKINETICS

Oxaliplatin is primarily eliminated in the urine. Renal clearance of platinum significantly correlates with glomerular filtration rate. The elimination half-life of oxaliplatin is about 70 hours.

DOSAGE AND SCHEDULE

Oxaliplatin has been administered as single agent therapy to heavily pretreated ovarian cancer patients on an every-3-week basis. In general, 59 to 130 mg/m^2 of oxaliplatin is administered as a 20-minute or 2-hour infusion. Oxaliplatin, like the other platinum agents, is highly emetogenic. Clearance of platinum is lower in patients with moderate renal impairment; however, no marked increase in drug toxicity has been noted. The effect of severe renal impairment on platinum clearance and toxicity is currently unknown. Oxaliplatin should not be given to patients with significant renal or hepatic dysfunction.

TOXICITY

HEMATOLOGIC

Unlike carboplatin, oxaliplatin produces only mild to moderate myelosuppression

GASTROINTESTINAL

Diarrhea
Vomiting
Mucositis

HEPATIC

Transaminase elevation

NEUROLOGIC

The main cumulative dose-limiting toxicity of oxaliplatin is peripheral sensory neuropathy

▆▆▆ Chlorambucil (Leukeran)

CHEMISTRY

Chlorambucil is a benzene butanoic acid derivative of nitrogen mustard with the chemical name 4-[bis(2-chloroethyl)amino] benzenebutanoic acid. Structurally, it is similar to melphalan. The chemical structure of chlorambucil is shown in Fig. 2.11.

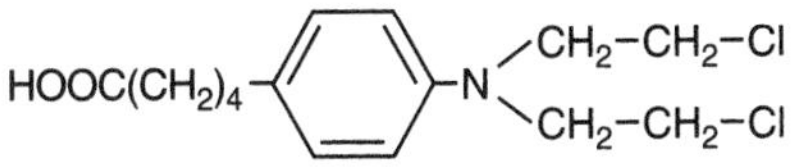

Figure 2.11.
Chemical structure of chlorambucil.

MECHANISM OF ACTION

Chlorambucil is a bifunctional alkylating agent. Its mechanism of action is typical for the alkylating agents. Central to its antitumor activity is the formation of DNA adducts.

CLINICAL PHARMACOLOGY AND PHARMACOKINETICS

Chlorambucil is rapidly and nearly completely absorbed (85%–90%) from the gastrointestinal tract after oral administration. Maximal plasma concentrations are reached in 40 to 70 minutes. The drug is almost completely metabolized by the liver. Some metabolites remain active. The primary active metabolite is phenylacetic acid mustard. Less than 1% of an oral dose is excreted in the urine as unchanged drug. The overall half-life of elimination is 1 or 2 hours.

DOSAGE AND SCHEDULES

When given for recurrent or persistent epithelial ovarian cancer:

> *Chlorambucil:* 0.1 to 0.2 mg/kg PO daily for 2 or 3 weeks
> *Chlorambucil:* 0.2 mg/kg PO daily for 5 days; repeat every 14 to 21 days

TOXICITY

HEMATOLOGIC

Myelosuppression: leukopenia and thrombocytopenia (may be cumulative and dose limiting)
Secondary malignancy (leukemia)

GASTROINTESTINAL

Nausea/vomiting
Diarrhea

Dermatologic
Alopecia (uncommon)

Hepatic
Increased SGOT (mild and transient)

Pulmonary
Pulmonary fibrosis (rare, may be cumulative)

Neurologic
Seizures (more common in the setting of renal insufficiency)
Peripheral neuropathy (rare)

■ ■ ■ Altretamine (Hexalen, hexamethylmelamine)

CHEMISTRY

Altretamine is an agent that also been referred to as hexamethylmelamine, Hexalen, NSC-13875, or simply HMM. It consists of a symmetric six-member triazene ring with three attached dimethylamine groups. Its chemical name is 2,4,6-tris (dimethylamine)-S-triazine. The chemical structure of altretamine is shown in Fig. 2.12.

MECHANISM OF ACTION

While altretamine shares chemical properties with alkylating agents, its mechanism of action remains uncertain. Altretamine does not display clinical cross-resistance with other alkylating agents, implying an alternative mechanism of action. The active intermediate species has not been identified.

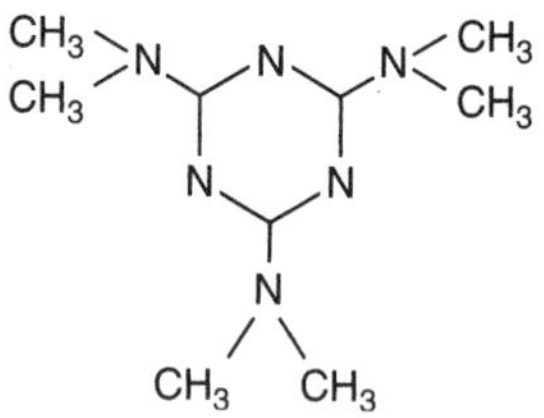

Figure 2.12.
Chemical structure of altretamine.

CLINICAL PHARMACOLOGY AND PHARMACOKINETICS

Altretamine has limited aqueous solubility and is therefore not given intravenously. It is well absorbed after oral administration (75%–90%). Peak plasma levels are achieved in 0.5 to 3 hours. There is an extensive first-pass effect in the liver. The microsomal P-450 enzymes metabolize altretamine to methylated metabolites. Less than 1% of altretamine is excreted unchanged in the urine. Drugs that modulate the liver microsomal enzymatic pathways may alter the half-life of altretamine. Phenobarbital would shorten and cimetidine would prolong the half-life of altretamine.

DOSAGE AND SCHEDULES

When given as a single agent for persistent or recurrent epithelial ovarian cancer:

> *Regimen 1:* 150 to 260 mg/m^2 altretamine PO daily for 14 days; cycles repeated every 28 days
> *Regimen 2:* 4 to 12 mg/kg altretamine PO daily for 14 to 21 days; repeat every 6 weeks

TOXICITY

HEMATOLOGIC

Myelosuppression: leukopenia and thrombocytopenia (nadir at 3 or 4 weeks with recovery within 2 or 3 weeks)
Secondary malignancies (leukemia)

GASTROINTESTINAL

Nausea/vomiting
Anorexia
Diarrhea

DERMATOLOGIC

Rash

NEUROLOGIC (FREQUENTLY DOSE LIMITING)

Paresthesias
Hyperesthesia
Hyperreflexia
Motor weakness

Decreased proprioception
Hallucinations
Confusion
Lethargy
Agitation
Depression
Ataxia
Coma

▬ *Antitumor Antibiotics*

Antitumor antibiotics are a class of chemotherapeutic agents that are generally derived from microorganisms. Most of these compounds have been isolated from fermentation products from various fungi. It is thought that the fungi produce these agents in order to inhibit the growth of other nearby organisms that are competing for nutrients. Most of these agents produce cytotoxic effects via DNA intercalation. In general, they are cell-cycle nonspecific. Mitoxantrone is a synthetic anthracycline analog that has been included in this class of agents.

▬ Dactinomycin (actinomycin D)

CHEMISTRY

Dactinomycin (actinomycin D) is composed of a central tricyclic phenoxazone chromophore that is linked to two identical cyclic polypeptides. The phenoxazone ring gives the drug its red-yellow color. It is a fermentation product of various Streptomyces species. Dactinomycin is produced for clinical use from *Streptomyces parvulus*. The chemical structure of dactinomycin is shown in Fig. 2.13.

MECHANISM OF ACTION

The cytotoxic effects of dactinomycin are the result of DNA intercalation. This leads to inhibition of DNA transcription and RNA translation. The phenoxazone ring structure intercalates between base pairs. The intercalation occurs most frequently at guanine residues. The two polypeptide rings of

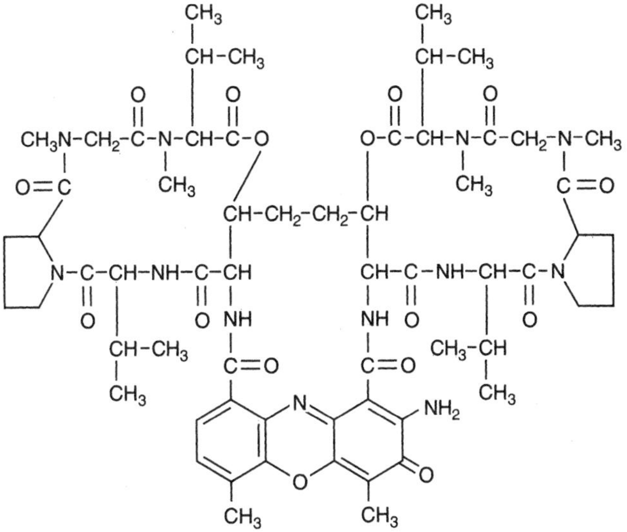

Figure 2.13.
Chemical structure of dactinomycin.

dactinomycin are then able to lie in the minor groove of DNA, which likely contributes to inhibition of DNA-directed RNA synthesis.

CLINICAL PHARMACOLOGY AND PHARMACOKINETICS

The clinical pharmacology of dactinomycin is poorly understood. It is poorly absorbed via the gastrointestinal tract. However, after intravenous administration, it is rapidly cleared from the plasma because of uptake by tissue and DNA binding. Most of the drug is eventually excreted unchanged in the urine and bile. The terminal half-life of elimination is approximately 36 hours.

DOSAGE AND SCHEDULES

When given as part of the EMA-CO regimen (etoposide-methotrexate-dactinomycin and cyclophosphamide-vincristine) for high-risk gestational trophoblastic disease:

Dactinomycin: 0.5 mg i.v. bolus on day 1; repeat every 14 days

When given as a single agent for nonmetastatic gestational trophoblastic disease:

Regimen 1: 9 to 15 μg/kg dactinomycin i.v. daily for 5 days; repeat every 14 to 21 days
Regimen 2: 1.25 mg/m² dactinomycin i.v. every 14 days

TOXICITY

HEMATOLOGIC

Myelosuppression: leukopenia and thrombocytopenia (at 7–14 days after administration)

GASTROINTESTINAL

Nausea/vomiting: occurs 1 hour after dose and lasts several hours
Mucositis/stomatitis
Radiation-recall stomatitis and enteritis

DERMATOLOGIC

Alopecia (may include accessory body hair)
Erythema
Hyperpigmentation
Extravasation results in severe pain, necrosis, and sloughing
Radiation-recall dermatitis

HEPATIC

Increased SGOT (rare)

■■■■ **Bleomycin**

CHEMISTRY

Bleomycin is a mixture of polypeptide fermentation products from the fungus Streptomyces verticillus first described by Umezawa in 1966. The predominant species is the A_2 polypeptide, which has been well studied. The chemical structure of bleomycin A_2 and the less common B_2 is shown in Fig. 2.14.

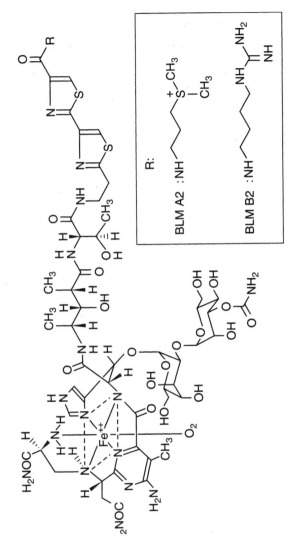

Figure 2.14.
Chemical structure of bleomycin.

MECHANISM OF ACTION

Bleomycin produces its cytotoxic effects via the induction of single-strand breaks in DNA. These effects are relatively DNA specific with only minor effects on RNA. This activity is dependent on the presence of a metal ion cofactor. Copper or iron ions as cofactors enable bleomycin to exert maximal cytotoxic effects. However, nickel, manganese, cobalt, and other metal ions are able to confer cytotoxicity to bleomycin. The metallic cofactor undergoes reduction, thereby gaining an electron. This promotes binding with oxygen and results in the formation of superoxide anions and hydroxy radicals, leading to DNA damage. The action of bleomycin appears to be cell-cycle specific for the G_2 phase.

CLINICAL PHARMACOLOGY AND PHARMACOKINETICS

Bleomycin is usually given intravenously However, it may be given subcutaneously or intramuscularly it is poorly absorbed from the gastrointestinal tract. The majority of the drug is excreted unaltered in the urine. Elimination from the plasma follows two-phase kinetics. The initial phase of elimination has a half-life of 24 minutes. The terminal phase of elimination has a half-life of 2 to 4 hours. It is very important to appropriately reduce the dosage in the setting of renal failure.

DOSAGE AND SCHEDULES

Note: Dosage expressed in units (1 U ≈ 1 mg bleomycin).

When given as part of the BEP regimen for ovarian germ cell tumors:

Bleomycin: 30 U/m^2 i.v. weekly

When given as a single agent for advanced or recurrent squamous carcinoma of the vulva:

Bleomycin: 10 to 20 U/m^2 i.v. or i.m. once or twice weekly

When given as part of a multiple-drug regimen for advanced or recurrent squamous carcinoma of the vulva:

Bleomycin: 5 to 15 U/m^2 i.v. daily for 3 to 6 days

TOXICITY

HEMATOLOGIC
Myelosuppression: mild

GASTROINTESTINAL
Nausea/vomiting: mild
Anorexia

DERMATOLOGIC
Hyperpigmentation (common)
Pruritus
Hyperkeratosis
Alopecia
Rash
Skin peeling
Mucositis

PULMONARY
Interstitial pneumonitis
Pulmonary fibrosis

These toxicities may be severe and are dependent on cumulative dose. Incidence increases with lifetime dosages over 400 U. Exposure to high concentrations of oxygen also increases pulmonary toxicity.

HYPERSENSITIVITY
Anaphylactoid reactions (reported incidence: 1%–8%); seen with greatest frequency in lymphoma patients

OTHER
Fever (commonly seen associated with chills): seen within 4 to 10 hours of administration and lasts up to 12 hours

■■■ Doxorubicin (Adriamycin)

CHEMISTRY

Doxorubicin is an anthracycline composed of a tetracyclic chromophore, adriamycinone, that is linked to the amino sugar daunosamine via a glycosic bond. The adriamycinone ring structure gives the drug its characteristic deep red color. The chemical structure of doxorubicin is shown in Fig. 2.15.

MECHANISM OF ACTION

There are multiple mechanisms that account for the cytotoxic effects of doxorubicin. Among these are topoisomerase II inhibition, DNA intercalation, and free radical formation.

An important mechanism of action is topoisomerase II–dependent DNA fragmentation. Topoisomerase II is one of the enzymes controlling the degree of DNA supercoiling. The degree of supercoiling is critical to normal protein–DNA interactions and gene function. The anthracyclines appear to alter the function of topoisomerase II. The enzyme is able to form its normal protein-associated double-strand breaks; however, anthracyclines inhibit the religation of the broken strands. This leads to multiple double-strand breaks in DNA. The frequency of double-strand breaks is roughly proportional to the efficacy of doxorubicin.

The adriamycinone ring structure is able to intercalate between DNA base pairs. Intercalation distorts the double

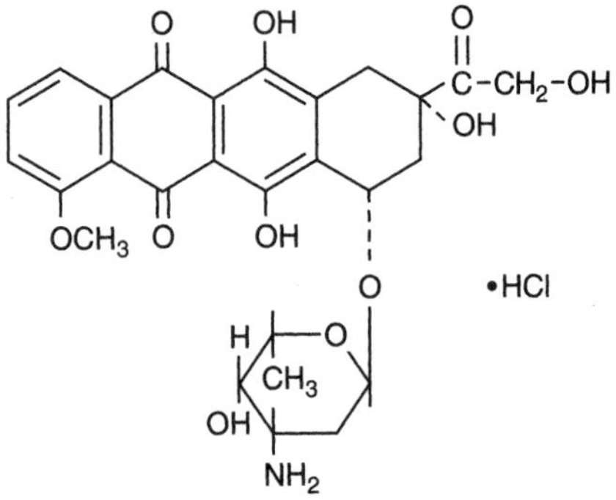

Figure 2.15.
Chemical structure of doxorubicin.

helix and contributes to inhibition of DNA-directed RNA synthesis. Additionally, intercalation probably triggers increased topoisomerase II activity, which increases the cytotoxic effects from inhibition of this enzyme by doxorubicin via an independent mechanism. Lastly, the daunosamine sugar side chain is able to lie in the minor groove of DNA, also contributing to inhibition of RNA synthesis.

A third potential mechanism of action of doxorubicin results from the formation of intracellular free radicals. The quinone group on the adriamycinone ring structure may undergo one-electron reduction to a semiquinone free radical. This unstable reduced state will rapidly donate the extra electron to molecular oxygen, resulting in restoration of the quinone and the formation of superoxide. The restored quinone may then again undergo redox cycling to produce more superoxide. The superoxide undergoes further reactions, forming hydrogen peroxide and a hydroxyl radical. Hydroxy radicals are highly reactive and may directly damage proteins, lipids, DNA, and RNA. It is likely that the formation of free radicals and the accumulation of hydrogen peroxide are the major contributors to the profound, dose-dependent cardiomyopathy observed with doxorubicin. Cardiac tissue has been shown to have particularly low levels of catalase, an important enzyme in the detoxification of hydrogen peroxide. These redox reactions are illustrated in Fig. 2.16.

CLINICAL PHARMACOLOGY AND PHARMACOKINETICS

Doxorubicin is approximately 70% protein bound after intravenous administration. It is not absorbed in significant amounts via the gastrointestinal tract. Therefore, oral administration is not indicated. The drug undergoes extensive hepatic metabolism to multiple products. The major active metabolite of doxorubicin is doxorubicinol. The parent drug and the metabolites are excreted in the urine and bile. The majority is cleared via the biliary route. Therefore, dose reduction of 50% to 70% is indicated in the setting of significant hepatic insufficiency (bilirubin ≥ 1.5). Doxoru-

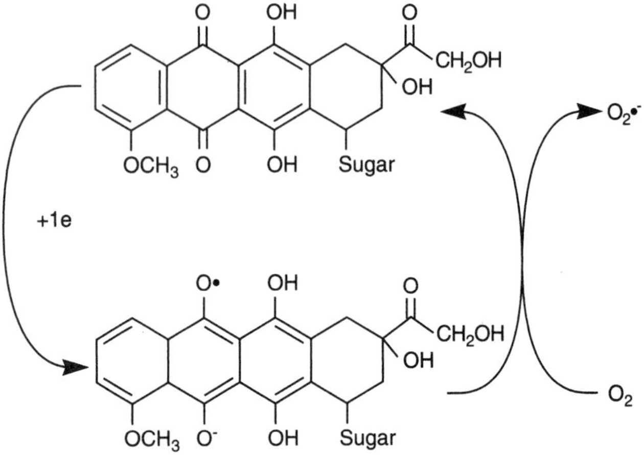

Figure 2.16.
Doxorubicin redox reactions.

bicin's half-life for elimination from the plasma is approximately 18 to 28 hours.

DOSAGE AND SCHEDULES

When given as part of a multidrug regimen for the treatment of ovarian, cervical, or endometrial cancer:

> *3-Week Regimen:* 60 to 75 mg/m^2 doxorubicin i.v. bolus every 3 weeks; do not exceed cumulative dose of 450 mg/m^2
>
> *Weekly Regimen:* 15 to 30 mg/m^2 doxorubicin i.v. bolus weekly; do not exceed cumulative dose of 450 mg/m^2

TOXICITY

HEMATOLOGIC

Myelosuppression: leukopenia (dose limiting) and thrombocytopenia (at 7–14 days after administration)

GASTROINTESTINAL

Nausea/vomiting
Mucositis/stomatitis

DERMATOLOGIC

Alopecia

Erythema

Hyperpigmentation

Extravasation results in severe pain, necrosis, and sloughing

Radiation-recall dermatitis (occasional)

CARDIAC

Cardiomyopathy leading to congestive heart failure. The incidence of this toxicity is dependent on cumulative dose as follows:

Cumulative Dose	Incidence of Cardiomyopathy
450 mg/m^2	3%
550 mg/m^2	7%
600 mg/m^2	15%
700 mg/m^2	40%

Preexisting cardiac disease or prior mediastinal radiation therapy may increase the dose-dependent incidence of cardiomyopathy.

Doxorubicin should be discontinued if left ventricular ejection fraction decreases by 10% or more associated with an absolute ejection fraction of less than 50%.

■ Liposomal doxorubicin HCl (Doxil)

CHEMISTRY

This chemotherapeutic agent is a liposomal formulation of doxorubicin. The chemical structure is shown in Fig. 2.17.

MECHANISM OF ACTION

Liposomal doxorubicin binds DNA and inhibits nucleic acid synthesis.

CLINICAL PHARMACOLOGY AND PHARMACOKINETICS

Liposomal doxorubicin has a small volume of distribution and has a much longer half-life compared with doxorubicin HCl. The percentage of this agent that is protein bound is unknown. The metabolite doxorubicinol is found in small

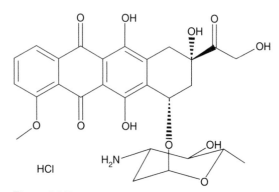

Figure 2.17.
Chemical structure of liposomal doxorubicin.

concentrations after the administration of liposomal doxorubicin in comparison with conventional doxorubicin.

DOSAGE AND SCHEDULE

The agent is commonly used as second line therapy for advanced ovarian cancer. The initial starting dosage of liposomal doxorubicin is as follows:

Liposomal doxorubicin: 50 mg/m^2 every 4 weeks

Dose reduction is required for hepatic insufficiency.

TOXICITY

HEMATOLOGIC
Myelosuppression: less severe than doxorubicin

GASTROINTESTINAL
Mild nausea/vomiting
Mucositis/stomatitis

DERMATOLOGIC
Hand and foot syndrome (palmar-plantar erythrodysesthesia): characterized by painful edema and erythema, which can be dose limiting

HYPERSENSITIVITY

Acute infusion-related reaction characterized by flushing, chills, back pain, shortness of breath, and hypotension has been reported in approximately 7% of patients; this reaction generally resolves within hours by either slowing down or discontinuing the infusion

CARDIAC

Cardiomyopathy is less common with liposomal doxorubicin compared with standard doxorubicin

■■ Mitomycin C

CHEMISTRY

Mitomycin C is a product of the fungus *Streptomyces caespitosus*. The molecule contains a quinone and an aziridine group. The chemical structure of mitomycin C is shown in Fig. 2.18.

MECHANISM OF ACTION

The cytotoxic effects of mitomycin C stem from its ability to act as an electron acceptor that contributes to the formation of alkylating groups. The alkylating properties allow for the formation of DNA adducts, resulting in inhibition of DNA synthesis. It appears that mitomycin C must participate in redox reactions to attain cytotoxic activity The quinone group accepts an electron, leading to the reduced semiquinone. This facilitates the opening of the aziridine ring, thereby creating alkylating groups. Additionally, the redox reactions result in the formation of toxic hydroxyl

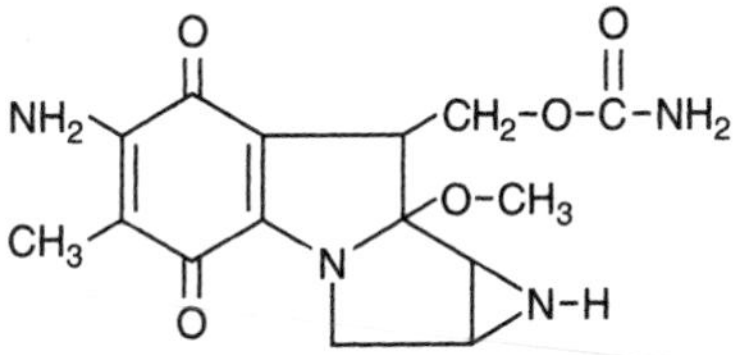

Figure 2.18.
Chemical structure of mitomycin C.

and superoxide radicals that may directly damage DNA, RNA, and cellular proteins. However, it is unclear to what extent the redox reactions contribute to the cytotoxicity of this drug. These reactions require an aerobic environment.

Once the alkylating groups are activated, mitomycin C has been shown to form DNA adducts at the O-6, N-7, and N-2 positions of guanine and the N-6 position of adenine.

CLINICAL PHARMACOLOGY AND PHARMACOKINETICS

Mitomycin C is poorly absorbed via the gastrointestinal tract and is therefore usually given intravenously. The drug is metabolized by the liver. Approximately 10% to 30% is excreted unchanged in the urine. The half-life for elimination from the plasma is 1 or 2 hours and may be prolonged in the setting of hepatic failure.

DOSAGE AND SCHEDULES

Mitomycin C: 10 to 20 mg/m^2 i.v. every 6 to 8 weeks

TOXICITY

HEMATOLOGIC

Myelosuppression: leukopenia and thrombocytopenia (nadir at 4 or 5 weeks with recovery lasting 2 or 3 weeks)
Hemolytic uremia syndrome may occur months after mitomycin C administration

GASTROINTESTINAL

Nausea/vomiting
Anorexia

DERMATOLOGIC

Alopecia
Erythema
Extravasation, resulting in severe pain, necrosis, and sloughing

HEPATIC

Venoocclusive disease of the liver

RENAL

Nephrotoxicity

Interstitial pneumonitis

Fatigue
Paresthesias

■■ Mitoxantrone

CHEMISTRY

Mitoxantrone contains a planar tricyclic anthraquinone ring structure. It is a completely synthetic anthracycline analog. It has the chemical name 1,4-dihydroxy-5,8-bis [[2-[(2-hydroxyethyl) amino] ethyl] amino]-9,10-anthracenedione dihydrochloride. The chemical structure of mitoxantrone is shown in Fig. 2.19.

MECHANISM OF ACTION

Mitoxantrone, like the anthracyclines, is a DNA-intercalating agent that undergoes reduction to a semiquinone. However, the mitoxantrone semiquinone is not reactive. This results in reduced cardiotoxicity when compared with doxorubicin. Most of the antitumor effect of mitoxantrone is probably mediated through the inhibition of topoisomerase II activity.

CLINICAL PHARMACOLOGY AND PHARMACOKINETICS

After intravenous administration, mitoxantrone is widely distributed. It is partially metabolized in the liver. The re-

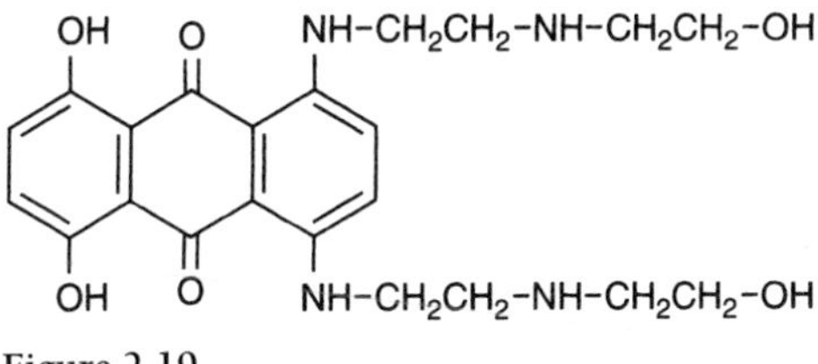

Figure 2.19.
Chemical structure of mitoxantrone.

mainder is excreted unchanged in the bile and urine. Studies have suggested that intraperitoneal administration of mitoxantrone may lead to persistence of active drug in the peritoneal cavity for 6 to 22 weeks.

DOSAGE AND SCHEDULES

When given for persistent epithelial ovarian carcinoma:

Mitoxantrone: 12 to 14 mg/m^2 i.v. every 3 weeks

For small-volume persistent ovarian carcinoma:

Mitoxantrone: 10 mg i.p. every 3 weeks

TOXICITY

HEMATOLOGIC
Myelosuppression: leukopenia and thrombocytopenia

GASTROINTESTINAL
Nausea/vomiting
Diarrhea
Abdominal pain (after IP administration)

DERMATOLOGIC
Alopecia
Blue discoloration of tissues (particularly sclerae)

HEPATIC
Transient elevations of hepatic transaminases

CARDIOVASCULAR
Congestive heart failure secondary to cumulative cardiomyopathy

NEUROLOGIC
Headache/seizures (rare)

■■■ *Agents Derived from Plants*

Several useful cytotoxic agents are derived from plants. A common theme in the cytotoxic activity of these agents is disturbance of normal assembly, disassembly, and stabilization of intracellular microtubules. Microtubules are present in all eukaryotic cells and play a critical role in cellular transport and maintenance of cell shape.

The vinca alkaloids, epipodophyllotoxins, and taxanes are naturally occurring substances isolated from plants. The vinca alkaloids are derived from the common periwinkle plant known as *Catharanthus roseus*. The epipodophyllotoxins are semisynthetic cytotoxic agents derived from the roots and rhizomes of the mandrake plant, *Podophyllum peltatum*. The taxanes are derived from the bark of *Taxus brevifolia* (paclitaxel) and *Taxus baccata* (Taxotere).

▬▬ Vinblastine (Velban), Vincristine (Oncovin), and Vinorelbine (Navelbine)

CHEMISTRY

Vincristine, vinblastine, and vinorelbine as a group are known as the vinca alkaloids, the latter compound being a semisynthetic derivative of vincristine. They are dimeric alkaloids that contain two linked multiring structures, vindoline and catharanthine. Vinblastine and vincristine are very similar in structure but have strikingly different chemotherapeutic effects and toxicity spectrums. Structurally, they differ only by the presence of a methyl group (vinblastine) or a formyl group (vincristine) on the vindoline nucleus. In contrast, the catharanthine unit is the site of structural modification in vinorelbine. The chemical structures of all vinca alkaloids are shown in Fig. 2.20.

MECHANISM OF ACTION

The vinca alkaloids inhibit normal microtubular polymerization by binding to the tubulin subunit at a site distinct from the taxane-binding site. The predominant cytotoxic effect appears to result from mitotic arrest by inhibiting formation of the mitotic spindle. However, it is likely that the inhibition of microtubular assembly contributes to the cytotoxic effects on cells that are not undergoing mitosis.

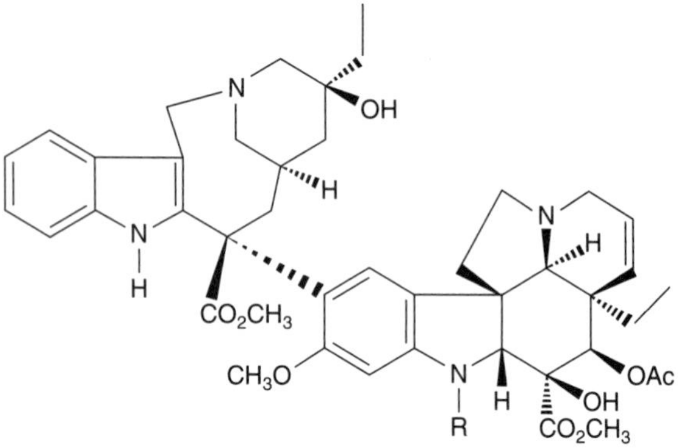

vincristine
R = CHO

vinblastine
R = CH₃

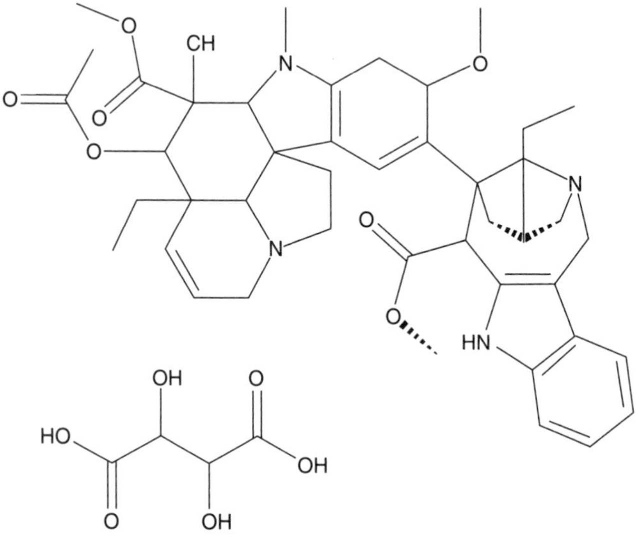

Vinorelbine tartrate

Figure 2.20.
Chemical structures of vinblastine, vincristine, and vinorelbine.

CLINICAL PHARMACOLOGY AND PHARMACOKINETICS

The vinca alkaloids are poorly absorbed by the gastrointestinal tract. They are all extensively bound to serum proteins. The predominant mechanism for elimination is via hepatic metabolism and biliary excretion. Hepatic elimination of the vinca alkaloids may be inhibited by the *MDR1* gene mechanism. Patients with abnormal liver function tests should not receive vinca-derived drugs. All vinca alkaloids have three-phase elimination kinetics. The initial half-life is less than 5 minutes and is mostly accounted for by uptake by plasma proteins. The second phase lasts 50 to 150 minutes, and the terminal phase is 24 to 90 hours.

DOSAGE AND SCHEDULES

When given as a continuous infusion for metastatic breast cancer or germ cell tumors:

Vinblastine: 1.5 to 2.0 mg/m^2 i.v. daily for 5 days

When given as a bolus infusion for metastatic breast cancer or germ cell tumors:

Vinblastine: 4.5 mg/m^2 i.v. every 21 days

When given as part of the EMA-CO regimen (etoposide-methotrexate-dactinomycin and cyclophosphamide-vincristine) for high-risk gestational trophoblastic disease:

Vincristine: 1.0 mg/m^2 i.v. every 15 days; maximum dose 2.0 mg

When given as a single agent for the treatment of recurrent cervical or ovarian cancer:

Vinorelbine: 20 to 30mg/m^2 every 1 or 2 weeks

TOXICITY

HEMATOLOGIC
Myelosuppression: leukopenia is dose limiting.

GASTROINTESTINAL
Nausea/vomiting (rare)
Abdominal cramps
Severe obstipation (vinblastine only)

DERMATOLOGIC

Vinblastine

Alopecia

Extravasation, resulting in severe pain, necrosis, and sloughing

Rash

Photosensitivity

Vincristine

Alopecia (common, up to 50%)

Extravasation, resulting in severe pain, necrosis, and sloughing

Vinorelbine

Alopecia

Extravasation, resulting in severe pain, necrosis, and sloughing

HEPATIC

Vincristine

SGOT and SGPT elevation (mild and transient)

NEUROLOGIC

Peripheral neuropathy

Autonomic neuropathy

Headache

Seizures

Cortical blindness (vincristine only)

PULMONARY

Bronchospasm (rare)

HYPERSENSITIVITY

Anaphylactoid reactions (reported incidence: 1%–8%); seen with greatest frequency in lymphoma patients

OTHER

Joint pain (especially the TMJ) after injection

SIADH

■■■ Etoposide (VP-16)

CHEMISTRY

Etoposide is produced as a glycosidic derivative of podophyllotoxin, produced in small amounts by the mandrake plant (*P. peltatum*). The structure of etoposide is characterized by a multiringed epipodophyllotoxin group bound to a glucopyranoside sugar. The chemical structure of etoposide is shown in Fig. 2.21.

MECHANISM OF ACTION

Like the vinca alkaloids, etoposide binds to the microtubular subunit tubulin. However, it is unclear what role inhibition of microtubular assembly plays in the overall cytotoxicity of etoposide. It is likely that the predominant cytotoxic effects of etoposide stem from interference with the normal functioning of topoisomerase II by stabilizing the putative cleavable enzyme–DNA complex in a cleavable state. This would promote the formation of single- and double-strand breaks in DNA, thereby contributing to cell death. Additionally, etoposide acts on topoisomerase II by interfering with normal "strandpassing," therefore altering the degree of supercoiling in DNA. These alterations in the degree of coiling of DNA may have profound effects on the efficiency of transcription and lead to cell death.

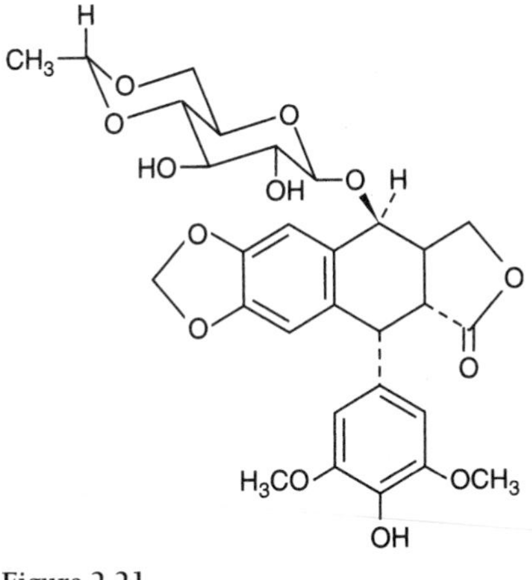

Figure 2.21.
Chemical structures of etoposide.

CLINICAL PHARMACOLOGY AND PHARMACOKINETICS

Etoposide is reasonably well absorbed via the gastrointestinal tract. However, absorption is variable among individual patients (25%–75%). It is extensively bound to plasma proteins. Etoposide is predominantly eliminated in the urine as unmetabolized drug. Approximately 10% to 15% is eliminated in the bile and passed in the feces. Elimination of etoposide follows biphasic kinetics. The initial half-life is approximately 1.5 hours and a terminal half-life is approximately 3 to 11 hours.

DOSAGE AND SCHEDULES

When given as part of the EMA-CO regimen (etoposide-methotrexate-dactinomycin and cyclophosphamide-vincristine) for high-risk gestational trophoblastic disease:

Day 1: 100 mg/m^2 etoposide i.v. bolus over 30 minutes.
Day 2: 100 mg/m^2 etoposide i.v. bolus over 30 minutes; repeat every 15 days

When given for advanced epithelial ovarian carcinoma:

Etoposide: 50 to 100 mg PO daily for 21 days; repeat cycles every 28 days

When given for ovarian germ cell tumors as part of the BEP regimen:

Etoposide: 100 mg/m^2 i.v. bolus over 30 minutes on days 1 through 5; repeat every 21 days

When given for uterine sarcomas:

Etoposide: 100 mg/m^2 i.v. bolus over 30 minutes daily for 3 days every 3 weeks

TOXICITY

HEMATOLOGIC

Myelosuppression: leukopenia (nadir at 7–14 days with recovery within 20 days)

GASTROINTESTINAL

Nausea/vomiting: common after oral administration
Anorexia

DERMATOLOGIC
Alopecia

HEPATIC
Hyperbilirubinemia (mild)
Increased transaminase levels (mild)

HYPERSENSITIVITY
Anaphylactoid reactions

CARDIOVASCULAR
Arrhythmias (rare)
Hypertension (rare, transient)

NEUROLOGIC
Peripheral neuropathy
Fatigue (rare)
Vertigo (rare)
Cortical blindness (rare, transient)

■■■ Paclitaxel (Taxol)

CHEMISTRY

Paclitaxel has a complex chemical structure composed of a 15-membered taxane ring system with an attached ester side chain at the C-13 position. The chemical structure of paclitaxel is shown in Fig. 2.22.

MECHANISM OF ACTION

Paclitaxel is an extract from the bark of the Western yew tree, *T. brevifolia*. It was first shown to have antitumor activity in the 1960s. It is believed that the C-13 ester side-chain is essential for antitumor activity. It binds to and stabilizes intracellular microtubules. The binding site for paclitaxel is distinct from the vinca alkaloid site. The stabilizing effect on microtubules occurs *in vitro* at concentrations as low as 0.05 μmol/L. At the cellular level, exposure to paclitaxel induces abnormal spindle formations that probably lead to the cytotoxic effect.

CLINICAL PHARMACOLOGY AND PHARMACOKINETICS

Paclitaxel is poorly soluble in aqueous solution. Therefore, it requires Cremophor EL and dehydrated alcohol USP as a

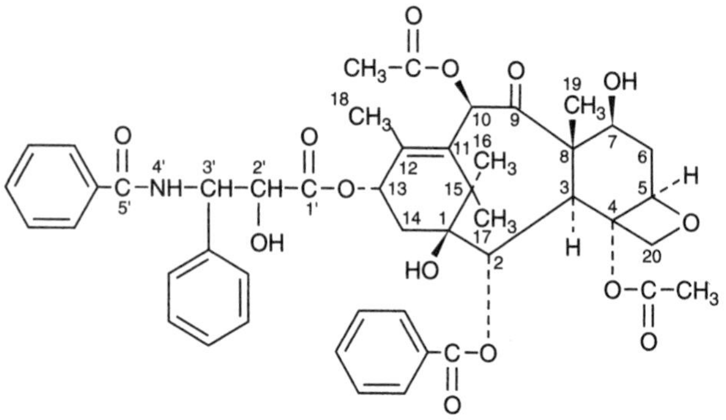

Figure 2.22.
Chemical structure of paclitaxel.

solvent. Even in Cremophor, precipitate may still be present, necessitating the use of a filter in the intravenous line. During a continuous intravenous infusion lasting 3 to 6 hours at standard doses, plasma concentrations of 1.3 to 13.0 pmol have been achieved. Over 95% of circulating paclitaxel is bound to plasma proteins. The elimination of paclitaxel follows nonlinear kinetics with an overall half-life of elimination ranging between 5 and 52 hours for a 24-hour infusion. If cisplatin is given immediately before paclitaxel in combination regimens, the elimination half-life of paclitaxel is prolonged. Although the exact mechanisms for the clearance of paclitaxel are not completely understood, hepatic metabolism by P-450 enzymes and biliary excretion are important. Animal studies have demonstrated that up to 42% of an injected dose is eliminated as metabolites and unchanged drug in the bile.

DOSAGE AND SCHEDULES

When given for epithelial ovarian cancer:

> *3-Hour Regimen:* 175 to 250 mg/m^2 i.v. over 3 hours every 3 weeks
> *24-Hour Regimen:* 135 to 175 mg/m^2 i.v. over 24 hours every 3 weeks

96-Hour Regimen: 120 to 140 mg/m^2 i.v. over 96 hours every 3 weeks

TOXICITY

HEMATOLOGIC

Myelosuppression: neutropenia (nadir at 8–11 days with recovery within 20 days; worse with longer infusion times)

GASTROINTESTINAL

Mucositis (worse with longer infusion time)

Nausea/vomiting (uncommon)

DERMATOLOGIC

Alopecia, including accessory hair (all patients, occurs 14–21 days after first dose)

HYPERSENSITIVITY

Flushing

Hypotension

Urticaria

Abdominal pain

Premedication with steroids and antihistamines (H$_1$ and H$_2$ blockers) recommended

CARDIOVASCULAR

Bradycardia (40–60 beats/min is common)

Ventricular tachycardia

Myocardial infarction (rare)

NEUROLOGIC

Peripheral neuropathy (more frequent with shorter infusion times and doses above 200 mg/m^2)

Fatigue (rare)

Headache

▬▬ Docetaxel (Taxotere)

CHEMISTRY

Docetaxel is a semisynthetic analogue of paclitaxel, prepared from a noncytotoxic precursor extracted from the needles of the European yew tree *T. baccata*. Its chemical name is N-debenzoyl-N-tert-butoxycarbonyl-10-deacytyl paclitaxel. The chemical structure of docetaxel is shown in Fig. 2.23.

MECHANISM OF ACTION

The antitumor effects of docetaxel occur via a similar mechanism to paclitaxel. Docetaxel promotes assembly and inhibits depolymerization of intracellular micro-tubules.

CLINICAL PHARMACOLOGY AND PHARMACOKINETICS

In animal studies, docetaxel has a broad spectrum of anti-tumor activity against a variety of transplantable human tumors. *In vitro* cytotoxicity assays suggest that it is two to five times more potent than paclitaxel. Pharmacokinetics of elimination of docetaxel between doses of 20 mg/m^2 and 115 mg/m^2 are linear. At higher doses, triphasic elim-ination has been observed. Excretion of unchanged drug in the urine is low (approximately 5% of administered dose).

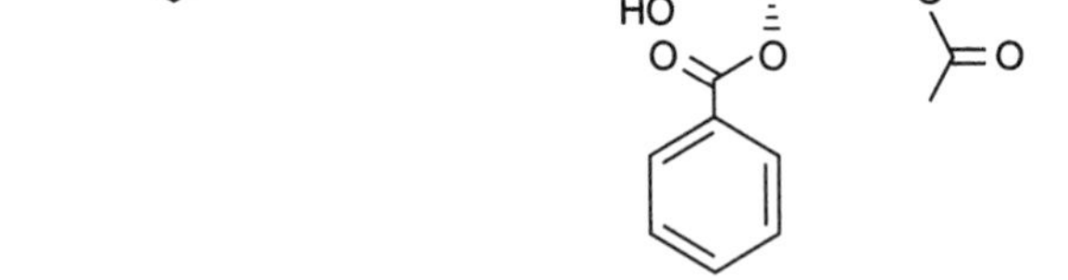

Figure 2.23.
Chemical structure of docetaxel. Reproduced with permission from Lavelle F: *Semin Oncol* 1995; 22(suppl 4):4.

DOSAGE AND SCHEDULES

When given for epithelial ovarian cancer (as a single agent or in combination with carboplatin)

Docetaxel: 60–100 mg/m² i.v. over 1 hour every 3 weeks

TOXICITY

HEMATOLOGIC

Myelosuppression: neutropenia

GASTROINTESTINAL

Mucositis

DERMATOLOGIC

Alopecia

HYPERSENSITIVITY

Flushing
Hypotension
Urticaria
Abdominal pain
Premedication with steroids and diphenhydramine recommended

CARDIOVASCULAR

Fluid retention
Serositis

▬ Topotecan (Hycamtin)

CHEMISTRY

Topotecan is a water-soluble analog of camptothecin, a multiringed plant product extracted from the wood stem of the Chinese tree *Camptotheca acuminata*. The parent compound was identified in the 1950s, but development was stymied by the insoluble nature of the compound and unpredictable toxicity. The unique mechanism of camptothecin supported continued interest and a variety of promising analogs have now entered clinical trials. The chemical structure of topotecan and irinotecan are shown in Fig. 2.24.

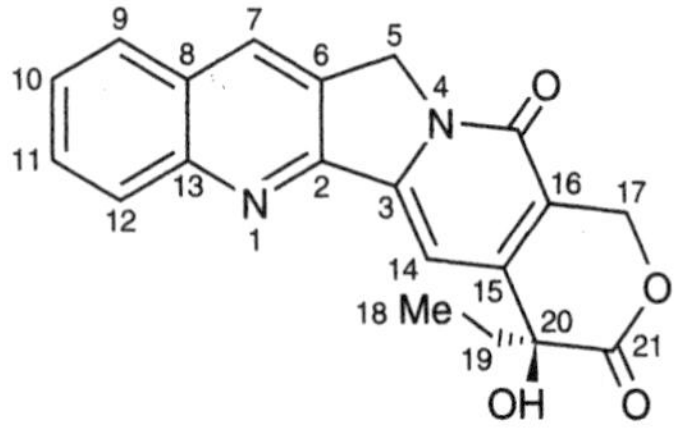

Substitutions:

Compounds	Position		
	7	9	10
Topotecan	H	$-CH_2-N\overset{CH_3}{\underset{CH_3}{}}$	$-OH$
Irinotecan (CPT-11)	$-CH_2-CH_3$	H	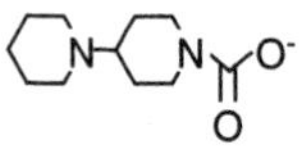 (piperidine ring)

Figure 2.24.
Chemical structure of topotecan and irinotecan.

MECHANISM OF ACTION

The mechanism of topotecan is thought to depend primarily on the inhibition of the nuclear enzyme topoisomerase I. When topotecan binds to topoisomerase I, single-stranded DNA breaks appear due to stabilized covalent bonds between genomic DNA and the topo I enzyme.

CLINICAL PHARMACOLOGY

The lactone ring of topotecan appears to be necessary for activity, and at higher pH conditions, the lactone ring opens to form an inactive hydroxyl form. The two forms appear to be in equilibrium in the body after administration. The drug is eliminated by active biliary transport and approximately one half of the administered dose will appear in the urine over the next 24 hours. The elimination half-life of topotecan is short, ranging from 1.7 to 4.9 hours, depending on the schedule of administration.

DOSAGE AND SCHEDULES

The optimal dose and schedule of topotecan remains an active area of clinical investigation. Early trials suggest that some ovarian cancers refractory to cisplatin and paclitaxel may respond to topotecan.

Daily × 5: 1.0–1.5 mg/m^2 i.v. over 30 min qd × 5
Weekly: 4 mg/m^2 i.v. day 1 and day 8; repeat every 21 days
   (investigational)

TOXICITY

Myelosuppression is the dose-limiting toxicity
Neutropenia greater than thrombocytopenia
G-CSF does not significantly increase tolerated dose

GASTROINTESTINAL
Nausea and vomiting (mild to moderate)
Diarrhea
Mucositis

SKIN
Alopecia
Rash

■■■ Irinotecan (CPT-11)

CHEMISTRY

Irinotecan is a water-soluble analog of camptothecin, a multiringed plant product extracted from the wood stem of the Chinese tree *C. acuminata*. The parent compound was identified in the 1950s, but development was stymied by the insoluble nature of the compound and unpredictable toxicity. The unique mechanism of camptothecin supported continued interest and a variety of promising analogs have now entered clinical trials. The chemical structure of irinotecan is shown in Fig. 2.24.

MECHANISM OF ACTION

The mechanism of irinotecan is thought to depend primarily on the inhibition of the nuclear enzyme topoisomerase I. When irinotecan binds to topoisomerase I, single-stranded DNA breaks appear due to stabilized covalent bonds between genomic DNA and the topo I enzyme.

CLINICAL PHARMACOLOGY

Irinotecan appears to have its clinical activity primarily through its hepatic metabolism (deesterification) to the highly active metabolite SN-38. SN-38 may be reformed in the gut after glucouronidation of the parent compound. The amount of SN38 in the gut lumen may correlate with the diarrhea associated with the drug. The pharmacology of irinotecan is complex and still poorly understood.

DOSAGE AND SCHEDULES

When given for the treatment of epithelial ovarian cancer:

Irinotecan: 300 mg/m^2 i.v. every 3 weeks or 100 mg/m^2 weekly for 4 weeks every 6 weeks

TOXICITY

HEMATOLOGIC

Myelosuppression is the dose-limiting toxicity
Neutropenia greater than thrombocytopenia
G-CSF does not significantly increase tolerated dose

GASTROINTESTINAL

Diarrhea can be severe and often dose limiting
Mucositis
Nausea and vomiting

SKIN

Alopecia
Rash

■■■ *Hormonal Agents*

Hormonal therapy is used for the treatment of endometrial, ovarian, and breast cancers. These agents may be broken into two classes: progestational agents and estrogen antagonists. Frequently used progestational agents include megestrol acetate (Megace), medroxyprogesterone acetate (Provera, Depo-Provera), and hydroxyprogesterone (Delalutin). Tamoxifen citrate (Nolvadex) is a frequently used antiestrogen.

▬ Megestrol acetate (Megace)

CHEMISTRY

Megestrol acetate is a synthetic progestational drug with antineoplastic activity It has the chemical name 17a-acetyloxy-6methyl-pregna-4,6-diene-3,20-diene.

MECHANISM OF ACTION

The mechanism by which megestrol acetate produces antineoplastic effects against breast and endometrial carcinoma is not well understood. However, inhibition of the production of pituitary gonadotropin leading to decreased estrogen secretion may be a factor. In addition, there may be a direct antineoplastic effect on breast and endometrial cancer cells. Other mechanisms of action have been suggested. It is possible that megestrol acetate interferes with the normal recycling of estrogen receptors on the cell surface, thereby reducing the number of available estrogen receptors. It also may interact directly with the genome to downregulate estrogen-responsive genes.

CLINICAL PHARMACOLOGY AND PHARMACOKINETICS

Megestrol acetate is variably absorbed after oral administration. Peak plasma concentrations are reached 1 to 3 hours after an oral dose. A small fraction of megestrol acetate is metabolized by the liver (5%–8%). Most of the drug is excreted unchanged in the urine (66%). The remainder is excreted unchanged in the feces (20%). The half-life of elimination from the plasma is variable, ranging from 13 to 105 hours (mean, 34 hours).

DOSAGE AND SCHEDULES

When given for palliative treatment of breast or endometrial carcinoma or endometrial stromal sarcoma:

Megestrol acetate: 40 mg PO qid

TOXICITY

GENERAL
Weight gain secondary to increased appetite

GASTROINTESTINAL
Nausea/vomiting (uncommon)

DERMATOLOGIC
Alopecia
Rash
Cushingoid facies

CARDIOVASCULAR
Thromboembolic phenomena
Thrombophlebitis
Hypertension

GYNECOLOGIC
Vaginal bleeding

▆▆▆ Tamoxifen citrate (Nolvadex)

CHEMISTRY

Tamoxifen citrate is a nonsteroidal, synthetic antiestrogen with the chemical name (Z)2-[4-(1,2-diphenyl-1-butenyl) phenoxy]N,N-dimethylethan-amine 2-hydroxy-1,2,3-propanetricarboxylate (1:1). It is a potent antiestrogen.

MECHANISM OF ACTION

Tamoxifen citrate is an estrogen antagonist. Its antitumor activity stems from the ability to compete with estradiol for binding to the estrogen receptor (ER). The tamoxifen–ER complex binding is reversible. The tamoxifen–ER complex is translocated to the nucleus where it reduces estrogen-mediated transcription and ultimately protein synthesis. The overall effect of tamoxifen is that of a cell cycle inhibitor, leading to the accumulation of cells in the G_0 and G_1 phases. Its effects are cytostatic (not cytocidal) and reversible upon cessation of the drug. Therefore, prolonged therapy with tamoxifen is often advocated.

CLINICAL PHARMACOLOGY AND PHARMACOKINETICS

Tamoxifen is well absorbed after oral administration. Peak plasma levels are reached 3 to 6 hours after an oral dose. Tamoxifen is extensively metabolized in the liver to multiple active and inactive compounds. The half-life of elimination of tamoxifen is approximately 7 days. The major active metabolite N-desmethyl tamoxifen is clinically relevant. This metabolite has a longer half-life (14 days) than the parent compound. Chronic administration leads to steady-state concentrations of N-desmethyl tamoxifen that are approximately twice that of the parent compound tamoxifen. This steady state develops after approximately 8 weeks of therapy.

DOSAGE AND SCHEDULES

When given for breast cancer:

Tamoxifen citrate: 10 mg PO bid

When given for ovarian cancer:

Tamoxifen citrate: 20 mg PO bid

TOXICITY

HEMATOLOGIC

Myelosuppression: thrombocytopenia (mild, transient), leukopenia (infrequent)

GASTROINTESTINAL

Nausea/vomiting (uncommon)
Anorexia (rare)
Diarrhea (rare)

DERMATOLOGIC

Rash (rare)
Erythema (rare)
Alopecia (rare)

HEPATIC

Increased transaminase levels (rare)
Cholestasis (rare)

GYNECOLOGIC

Secondary malignancies (endometrial carcinoma)
Endometrial polyps
Menstrual irregularities
Vulvar pruritus
Abnormal vaginal bleeding

CARDIOVASCULAR

Hot flushes (common)
Thrombophlebitis
Thromboembolism
Pulmonary embolism

NEUROLOGIC

Dizziness (rare)
Headache (rare)
Confusion (rare)

OCULAR

Retinopathy (rare)
Decreased visual acuity (rare)
Cataracts (rare)
Optic neuritis (rare)

GENERAL

Tumor flare characterized by bone and/or soft-tissue pain
with occasional hypercalcemia during the first few weeks
of therapy

■■■ Monoclonal Antibody Therapy

■■■ Oregovamab (Ovarex) (Investigational)

CHEMISTRY

Oregovamab (Mab-B43.13) is a murine monoclonal antibody that binds with high affinity (1.16×10^{10} M^{-1}) to CA125.

MECHANISM OF ACTION

Oregovamab antitumor activity is thought to be mediated through presentation of MAb-B43.13-CA125 immune complexes, leading to induction of CA125-specific antibodies and T cells. T cell and humoral (HAMA-human anti-mouse antibody) responses to oregovamab therapy correlate with a significant increase in time to disease progression. Oregovamab was tested in patients with ovarian cancer with a complete clinical remission.

CLINICAL PHARMACOLOGY AND PHARMACOKINETICS

After intravenous administration, oregovamab forms a complex with CA125 antigen. These oregovamab–CA125 complexes enhance immune recognition of the antigen. This enhanced immune recognition is postulated to be due to (1) altered CA125 uptake by antigen presenting cells (APCs), (2) upregulation of co-stimulatory molecules on dendritic cells, (3) CA125 antigen presentation through HLA class I and II, and (4) activation of CD4 and CD8 T cell subsets specific for CA125 and autologous tumor.

DOSAGE AND SCHEDULE

Oregovamab: 2 mg i.v. every 4 weeks until relapse

TOXICITY

Toxicity profile was similar to placebo.

■■■ Cetuximab (IMC-C225) (Investigational)

CHEMISTRY

Cetuximab (IMC-C225) is a chimeric monoclonal antibody that binds selectively to the epidermal growth factor receptor (EGFR).

MECHANISM OF ACTION

Cetuximab is a chimeric monoclonal antibody that is directed against the extracellular domain of the EGFR. This agent also selectively inhibits activation of the EGFR tyrosine kinase. This interaction is thought to prevent EGFR-mediated growth signaling in cancer cells. This agent is also under clinical development in cancer patients. Recent studies have shown that cetuximab is active in combination with irinotecan in patients with irinotecan refractory colorectal cancer. Cetuximab has also been used in combination with radiation therapy for the treatment of head and neck cancer. Surprisingly, cetuximab appears to be equally effective in EGFR-overexpressing tumors and tumors that do not overexpress EGFR.

CLINICAL PHARMACOLOGY AND PHARMACOKINETICS

Cetuximab is administered intravenously. The elimination of cetuximab is not well established.

DOSAGE AND SCHEDULE

Cetuximab: 200 to 250 mg/m^2 i.v. weekly

TOXICITY

GASTROINTESTINAL
Nausea

DERMATOLOGIC
Acne-like rash

HYPERSENSITIVITY
Allergic reaction (fever, chills, erythema)

HEPATIC
Transaminase elevation

▬▬ Targeted Therapy

▬▬ Gefitinib (Iressa, ZD1839) (Investigational)

CHEMISTRY

The chemical structure of gefitinib is shown in Fig. 2.25.

MECHANISM OF ACTION

Gefitinib is an orally active, quinazolone derivative that selectively inhibits the EGFR tyrosine kinase. EGFR expression is increase on a number of human cancers and inhibition of the EGFR signaling pathway is thought to prevent an important growth signal in cancer cells. Gefitinib is a small

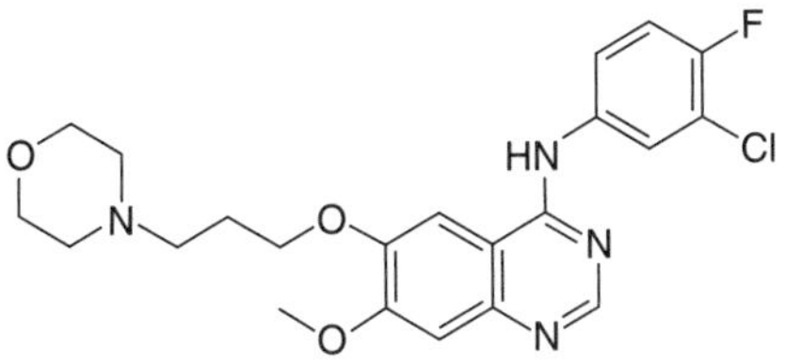

Iressa

Figure 2.25.
Chemical structure of gefitinib.

molecule inhibitor of the EGFR tyrosine kinase, and Iressa is under clinical development in cancer patients. *In vitro* and *in vivo* studies suggest that this agent has activity against ovarian cancer. Experimental models also suggest that gefitinib has synergy with other chemotherapeutic agents including paclitaxel, and also with radiation therapy. Phase 3 trials are underway combining gefitinib with gemcitabine, cisplatin, carboplatin, or paclitaxel.

CLINICAL PHARMACOLOGY AND PHARMACOKINETICS

It is unclear at this time how gefitinib is metabolized. Urinary recovery of the drug is minimal, suggesting that this is not the major route of elimination. The elimination half-life is 28 hours. A food-effect study showed that food intake with gefitinib did not affect the elimination half-life.

DOSAGE AND SCHEDULE

Iressa has been administered at a dosing schedule of 100 mg once daily for three days in early clinical trials. In the lung cancer trials daily doses of 250–500 mg were administered with carboplatin and paclitaxel. However, dose-limiting toxicity has not been reached with this dosing schedule.

TOXICITY

GASTROINTESTINAL

Diarrhea

Acne-form rash

▰▰▰ OSI-774 Erlotinib (Investigational)

CHEMISTRY

OSI-774 is an orally active small molecule inhibitor of the EGFR tyrosine kinase domain. This agent is currently in phase 2 trials in ovarian cancer.

MECHANISM OF ACTION

OSI-774 is a selective small molecule inhibitor of the EGFR tyrosine kinase domain (similar to gefitinib). The interaction of OSI-774 with the tyrosine kinase domain of the EGFR is thought to prevent EGFR-mediated growth signaling in cancer cells. Preliminary activity in ovary cancer has been observed.

CLINICAL PHARMACOLOGY AND PHARMACOKINETICS

OSI-774 is administered orally and continuously. The elimination of OSI-774 is not well established. The elimination half-life is 24 hours.

DOSAGE AND SCHEDULE

OSI-774: 150 mg/m^2 p.o. daily

TOXICITY

GASTROINTESTINAL
Diarrhea

DERMATOLOGIC
Acne-like rash

GENERAL
Fatigue
Headache

▰▰▰ Bortezomib (Velcade)

CHEMISTRY

Bortezomib is a small molecule that is a reversible proteosome inhibitor. The chemical structure is shown in Fig. 2.26.

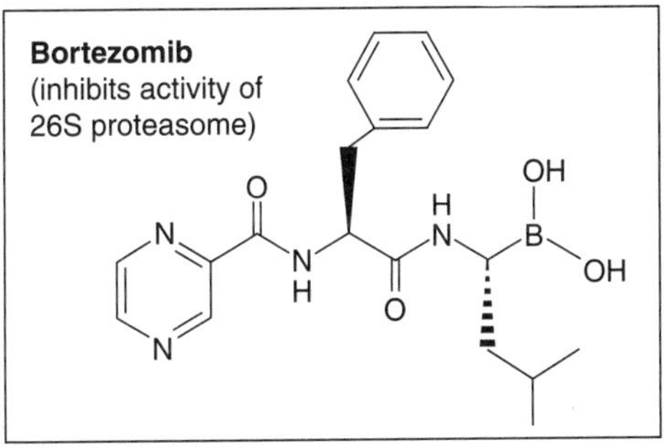

Figure 2.26.
Chemical structure of bortezomib.

MECHANISM OF ACTION

Bortezomib is a reversible inhibitor of the 26S proteosome, a multisubunit protein complex that is present in all cells and involved in protein degradation. Certain protein targets are those that are critical to regulation of the cell cycle, transcription and apoptosis. Nuclear factor-κ B (NF-κB) is a protein that, when activated, prevents cells from undergoing apoptosis. Its activity is in turn controlled by the inhibitor protein IκB, which is degraded by the 26S proteosome. Inhibition of IκB degradation therefore results in inhibition of NF-κB, thereby resulting in cell death. The inhibition of the 26S proteosome by bortezomib therefore leads to apoptosis.

CLINICAL PHARMACOLOGY AND PHARMACOKINETICS

Bortezomib is given intravenously. It has a high volume of distribution, and is over 80% bound to serum protein. Levels are rapidly cleared from the serum. Further pharmacokinetic data on Bortezomib in humans are not well established.

DOSAGE AND SCHEDULES

This is currently an investigational agent. Preliminary studies suggest activity in epithelial ovarian cancer. Dosages below are based upon studies in patients with multiple myeloma

Bortezomib: 1 to 1.3 mg/m^2 i.v. twice a week × 2 to 4 weeks

TOXICITY

HEMATOLOGIC
Myelosuppression (mild)

GASTROINTESTINAL
Diarrhea
Nausea, vomiting
Abdominal distension

DERMATOLOGIC
Rash

HEPATIC
Elevation in SGOT/alkaline phosphatase

PULMONARY
Dyspnea

CARDIAC
Hypotension

NEUROLOGIC
Peripheral neuropathy (frequent)
Headache
Dizziness
Fatigue

OTHER
Fever
Myalgias/arthralgia

Selected Reading

Arky R: *Physician's Desk Reference*, 49th edition. Medical Economics, Montvale, NJ, 1995.

Calvert AH: Prospective evaluation of simple formula based on renal function. *J Clin Oncol* 1989; 7:1748–1756.

Chabner B, Longo D (eds): *Cancer Chemotherapy and Biotherapy. Principles and Practice*, 2nd edition. Lippincott, Philadelphia, 1996.

DeVita VT, Hellman S, Rosenberg SA: *Cancer: Principles and Practice of Oncology,* 4th edition. J. B. Lippincott, Philadelphia, 1993.

DiSaia PJ, Creasman WT: *Clinical Gynecologic Oncology*, 4th edition. Mosby-Year Book, St. Louis, 1993.

Fischer DS, Knobf MT, Durivage, HJ: *The Cancer Chemotherapy Handbook*, Mosby Year Book, St. Louis, 1993.

Hoskins WJ, Perez CA, Young RC: *Principles and Practice of Gynecologic Oncology*, 1st edition J. B. Lippincott, Philadelphia, 1992.

Perry MC: *The Chemotherapy Sourcebook*, 1st edition. Williams & Wilkins, Baltimore, 1992.

Rubin SC, Sutton GP: *Ovarian Cancer*, 1st edition McGraw-Hill, New York, 1993.

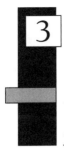

3

DESIGN OF CLINICAL TRIALS

JOHN BLESSING

A clinical trial has been defined as "a scientific experiment to generate clinical data for the purpose of evaluating one or more therapies on a population" (1). The appropriateness of the design will determine the scientific validity of the results. Inherent in the design are numerous issues including appropriate sample size, identification of the patient population, allocation of treatment, relevant parameters to judge outcome, ethical considerations, and proper interpretation. A brief introduction to each of these topics is provided in this chapter.

Study Design and Objectives

In order to investigate the efficacy of new therapies, several types of clinical trials have been devised. It is of critical importance to appreciate both the purpose and limitations of each. Additionally, it is essential that the objectives of the study be determined prior to the onset of the investigation. This is best accomplished in a multidisciplinary setting that fosters interaction between medical investigators and statisticians.

Phase 1 Study

Earliest indications of possible therapeutic efficacy typically result from animal or basic science studies. It is then necessary to conduct trials involving human subjects. The most

Chemotherapy of Gynecologic Cancers: Society of Gynecologic Oncologists Handbook 2e, edited by Stephen C. Rubin, MD, Lippincott Williams & Wilkins, Philadelphia © 2004.

elementary of these is the phase 1 trial, which attempts to determine a tolerable dose and schedule. At this level, no attempt is made to ascertain level of activity; the focus is to establish a maximum tolerated dose (MTD) that can be safely administered.

The phase 1 clinical trial does not lend itself to rigorous statistical analysis. Rather, a somewhat arbitrary, but nonetheless efficient, rule of thumb has emerged. An initial dose level is given to three consecutive patients. If no significant adverse effects are noted, the dose is raised to a higher level and three additional patients are treated. This procedure is continued until significant adverse effects are noted. At this time, the dose is reduced back to the previous level and an additional three patients are treated. If no significant toxicity occurs, this dose is declared to be the MTD and the trial is complete.

████ Phase 2 Study

Upon the determination of the MTD, a phase 2 trial may be initiated to obtain information regarding efficacy, which is typically measured by objective response rates and associated toxicity. The purpose of this trial is not to perform a definitive comparison with current standard therapy, but rather to identify therapeutic agents that might warrant further study in such a comparative trial.

The design of the phase 2 study must be well conceived for several reasons. Ethical considerations require that an undue number of patients must not be subjected to ineffective therapy; patient availability is a precious resource that cannot be squandered. However, sufficient patients must be treated to ensure that the results constitute more than a mere collection of anecdotes. Otherwise, minimally effective agents may be recommended for further study. Thus, sample size determination is critical.

In the past, the response rate has been estimated and confidence intervals have been constructed. More recently, two-stage designs employing stopping rules have been developed to optimize the number of patients required; this technique features a test of hypothesis regarding the true response rate. The null hypothesis is that the true response rate is less than some particular value, while the alternative is that it is greater than some larger value; for example, we might test the hypothesis that the true response rate is less than 10% versus the alternative hypothesis that it is greater than 30%. Both accrual and follow-up are divided into two stages. Following completion of the first stage, three outcomes are possible: If the number of observed responses is negligible, no further outcomes are possible. If the number of observed responses is particularly high, no further accrual is required and further testing is warranted. Finally, if the number of observed responses is intermediate, the second stage of accrual is required, followed by an additional test of the hypothesis; the specific stopping rules require the input of experienced statisticians.

Finally, the population studied must be homogeneous; the temptation to combine such disease entities as mixed mesodermal sarcomas and leiomyosarcomas or squamous cell and nonsquamous cell carcinomas of the cervix must be avoided.

■■■ Phase 3 Trial

Upon the completion of a phase 2 trial, the results may indicate that further investigation of the agent is warranted. This is typically true if the response rate appears to be potentially higher than that achieved with standard therapy A phase 3 study is a controlled randomized clinical trial whose primary purpose is to compare the efficacy of new regimens to standard therapy In any case, such a comparison must not be made on the basis of the observation of a phase 2 trial, but rather on the basis of an appropriately designed and conducted phase 3 study.

The design of a phase 3 study is a complex issue that cannot be addressed completely in this brief chapter. Of paramount importance is study feasibility, which is an intricate synthesis of medical relevance and mathematical limitations. Accordingly, it must be accomplished by sophisticated interaction of medical investigators and statisticians. An example of the complexity is seen in sample size determination for studies investigating response rates. Four key consideration areas are pivotal:

1. The magnitude of the therapeutic difference sought. (This will typically be 15%–20%. Larger differences require fewer patients, but are less likely to be realized.)
2. The response rate of the standard therapy (It is not intuitively obvious, but detection of a particular difference requires more patients if the response rate of the standard is near 50% than if it is at either extreme.)
3. The probabilities of false positive and false negative error rates that will be associated with the hypothesis testing involved in the comparison.
4. The nature of the alternative hypothesis. That is, does medical logic indicate the possibility that the new therapy could be inferior to the standard or do we only care if it is better. The former ("two-sided" alternative) requires more patients than the latter ("one-sided" alternative). The majority of clinical trials feature one-sided alternative hypotheses. An example of a design in which a one-sided alternative is appropriate is GOG Protocol 108, which is a randomized comparison of ifosfamide with or without cisplatin in patients with advanced, persistent, or recurrent mixed mesodermal tumors of the uterus. The schema for this study is depicted in Figure 3.1. It is not likely that the simple addition of cisplatin would lessen the response rate due to ifosfamide alone.

The combination of these four factors comprises the cornerstone of sample size determination. While no simplified formula can be presented for sample size determination, it is stressed that the number of cases required is sufficiently large that phase 3 trials are not generally practiced in a single clinical setting.

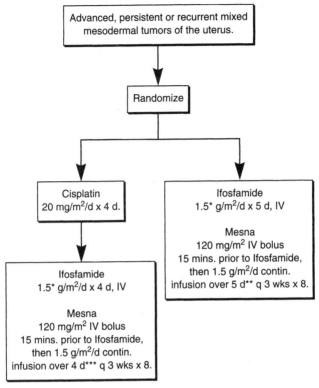

Figure 3.1.
GOG Protocol 108.

▄▄▄ *Eligibility*

The impact of a well-designed study is not restricted to those patients who received the therapy; indeed, the motivation for conducting such research is to enable appropriate inferences to be made regarding the population of patients with the same disease. Consequently, the precise definition of the population of interest is critical. In a clinical trial this is accomplished by delineating unambiguous and comprehensive eligibility criteria. Several eligibility criteria frequently employed in the investigation of gynecologic malignancies are briefly discussed.

▆▆▆ Performance Status

The Gynecologic Oncology Group (GOG) has employed a performance grade, based on the Karnofsky scale. In general, patients with performance status 0–2 are considered eligible. In this fashion, the results will not be enhanced by allowing only those patients with the best prognosis. Conversely, the therapy will be given an adequate test not compromised by extremely poor prognosis. It is important to establish a standard to ensure a level of compatibility.

▆▆▆ Site of Disease/Histology

Separate investigations of ovary, cervix, and corpus are mandated as each is a unique population of patients. However, it may not be as obvious that certain histologic types should also be treated as separate entities. The distinct combinations of site and histologic types most frequently studied separately are:

a. Epithelial ovarian carcinoma
b. Squamous cell carcinoma of the cervix
c. Nonsquamous cell carcinoma of the cervix
d. Endometrial carcinoma
e. Mixed mesodermal uterine sarcomas
f. Leiomyosarcoma of the uterus
g. Carcinoma of the vulva
h. Ovarian sarcomas
i. Trophoblastic disease

▆▆▆ Stage of Disease

The GOG employs the International Federation of Gynecology and Obstetrics (FIGO) staging nomenclature in clinical investigation of diseases from stage I to recurrent disease. Eligibility criteria must specify those stages of disease that are of interest. Many nuances exist; for example, in epithelial ovarian carcinoma, stage III optimal disease is generally investigated separately from stage III suboptimal disease. Thus, the amount of residual disease remaining after surgery is a consideration in establishing staging eligibility criteria.

▬ Prior Surgery

To address the staging and residual disease issues noted above, many studies require a specified surgical procedure at a minimum. Thus, the type of prior surgery is a consideration. Additionally, the timing of such surgery is a factor. While the patient must have recovered from the effects of surgery, the results of the surgery must still be relevant. Many studies require entry within 6 weeks of surgery for this reason.

▬ Prior Therapy

Decisions must be made as to what types of prior therapy will be allowed. Specific areas to consider are chemotherapy, radiotherapy, hormonal therapy, and immunotherapy These are not always simple issues. For example, if prior chemotherapy is allowed, will it be limited to one prior regimen or more? Also, is chemotherapy employed as a radiation sensitizer considered prior chemotherapy?

▬ Prior Malignancies

Generally speaking, patients who have had prior malignancies are not eligible for clinical trials.

▬ Pretreatment Blood Work and Laboratory Values

Levels required for eligibility must be determined.

▬ Measurable Disease

If measurable disease is required for response evaluation, criteria must be delineated not just for entry, but also to ensure the ability to obtain consistent follow-up measurements. Will CTs or chest x-rays be required?

The above discussion of common eligibility criteria is not exhaustive, and two other aspects must be emphasized: First, once the criteria are established, it is mandatory to adhere to them and not make exceptions. Second, in presenting the results, the eligibility factors must be explicitly noted in a "material and methods" section to ensure that the reader interprets the results correctly.

■■■■ Treatment Assignment: Randomization

Having ascertained patient eligibility, assignment of therapy is appropriate. To avoid any selection bias, it is essential that all eligible patients be entered. In the phase 2 setting only one therapy is typically involved and consequently this task is straightforward. In rare instances, randomized phase 1T trials are conducted to investigate two therapies simultaneously It is stressed that this randomization is merely to avoid investigator bias. It is used as method of entry and does not allow any comparisons of the two therapies.

In the phase 3 setting random allocation of treatment regimens is employed to allow meaningful comparisons to be made. This technique aims to create a situation in which observed differences will be due to the therapy and not due to the patient composition of the treatment arms. Randomization maximizes the opportunity for each regimen to feature comparable patients, although this cannot be guaranteed.

■■■■ Stratification

To further the likelihood that the regimens will be comparable with regard to prognostic factors, stratification is frequently employed. Prognostic variables are categorized at various "levels." Mutually exclusive subsets, called strata, are then defined by considering all possible combinations of these levels. Each stratum is randomized separately. For example, let us consider two prognostic variables, each with two levels: prior radiotherapy (yes versus no) and size of residual lesion (:5 2 cm versus > 2 cm). The resulting strata would then be:

- Prior radiotherapy, residual ≤2 cm
- Prior radiotherapy, residual >2 cm
- No prior radiotherapy, residual ≤2 cm
- No prior radiotherapy, residual >2 cm

Finally, it is noted that excessive stratification should be avoided. Otherwise, treatment balance within each of the large number of resulting strata will not be achieved.

■■■ Study Endpoints

The most frequently employed endpoints are adverse effects, response, progression-free survival, and survival. Recently efforts have been initiated to augment these quantitative measures with quality-of-life assessments. To achieve unambiguous results, these endpoints must be defined precisely.

■■■ Adverse Effects

Objective criteria are required to assess the severity of adverse effects associated with treatment. The Gynecologic Oncology Group has developed adverse effects criteria (2) for categorizing frequently encountered toxicity as none, mild, moderate, severe, or life-threatening. This enables otherwise subjective occurrences to be quantified. Moreover, it enables separate investigations to be evaluated in a standard fashion.

■■■ Response

Clinical response must also be categorized according to objective criteria. The GOG has delineated response. Of particular note is the fact that partial response requires each lesion followed to exhibit a 50% reduction. Here it is critical that one form of tumor measurement (physical exam, CT, chest x-ray) be consistently employed. Other methods to quantify response have been employed where appropriate. One such example is the use of second-look surgical procedures to classify response surgically.

■■■ Progression-free Survival and Survival

The GOG defines progression-free survival as date from entry to a particular protocol to date of reappearance or increasing parameters of disease, or to date of last contact. Survival is defined as observed length of life from entry to a particular protocol to death or, for living patients, date of last contact.

■■■ Quality of Life

Efforts to assess the effects of cancer and cancer therapy on the quality of the patient's life are also warranted. A wide variety of issues arise in this area. Methodology varies and is currently evolving. Difficulties that arise include "anything from the definition of the concept and constructing a questionnaire to the choice of method for calculations and analysis of the results" (3). Here again a multidisciplinary approach is warranted to ensure the input of ethicists and psychosocial experts.

■■■ *Early Stopping Rules*

Ethical practice requires the implementation of early stopping rules, where appropriate, to guarantee that patients are not unnecessarily subjected to inactive or inferior therapy In the phase 2 arena one such rule has already been described. In phase 3 studies, the design will typically specify one or two interim analyses during the study to accommodate such ethical considerations. However, numerous therapeutic comparisons are not appropriate as they would violate the underlying statistical principles inherent in the design. Both the number and timing of these analyses must be planned in advance.

▬▬ *Interpretation*

Several principles are noted regarding the proper interpretation of results. The purpose of this presentation is to introduce the notions. They cannot be thoroughly discussed in this brief section.

▬▬ Phase 2 Trials

It would be naive to think that subconscious comparisons to standard therapy will not occur. It is therefore crucial to remember that while such comparisons are necessary to determine if further investigation is warranted, they are also inconclusive. This limitation must be appreciated to avoid serious misinterpretation.

▬▬ "Negative" Studies

As noted in the Phase 3 Trials section, point 1, one of the factors inherently involved in study design is the magnitude of the difference in response rate, survival, etc., considered clinically significant to detect. If an appropriately designed comparative study does not proclaim such a difference, it is frequently considered to be a "negative" study This does not mean that there is "no difference" between the regimens. Rather, it implies that a difference of at least the magnitude considered clinically significant to detect in the design phase does not exist. Smaller differences may or may not exist. The study was not designed to investigate these smaller differences and therefore can offer no insight into this matter. (Recall that an investigation into smaller therapeutic differences would have required a greater sample size. Moreover, if a smaller difference was observed, it is inappropriate to enter additional cases in an effort to create statistical significance. The design phase may be thought of as similar to bidding in bridge. Once the hand is played, you cannot go back and rebid based on outcome.) For more information, see reference 4.

▰▰▰ Premature Analysis

Early results are based on a smaller number of cases and consequently the results are subject to considerable fluctuation. Apparent differences seen early in studies often disappear; initial estimates of response rates frequently bear no resemblance to those ultimately noted; "tails" of survival curves are based on a fraction of all patients entered and may change dramatically with very little change in data. For these reasons, data must not be analyzed earlier than planned for in study design. The consequences may be severe. Agents with little activity may be passed on to further study. Conversely, active agents may be overlooked. A more detailed presentation is found in Blessing and Anderson (5).

▰▰▰ *Conclusions*

In this chapter, several facets of clinical trials and design and conduct have been introduced. It is not practical or prudent to attempt a comprehensive discussion about them. Rather the intent is to create an awareness of the issues in the hopes that the clinical investigator will be a more discerning reader of articles and appreciate the value of medical-statistical interaction in conducting his or her own research.

References

1. Zelen M: Guidelines for publishing papers on clinical trials: Responsibilities of editors and authors. *J Clin Oncol* 1983; 1:164–169.
2. Blessing J: Design, analysis and interpretation of chemotherapy trials in gynecologic cancer. In G Deppe (ed.), *Chemotherapy of Gynecologic Cancer*. Alan R. Liss, New York, 1984, pp. 49–83.
3. Berger M: Quality of life, health status and clinical research. Med Care 1989; 3:148–156.
4. Blessing J: Biostatistics. In S Gusberg (ed.), *Female Genital Cancer*. Churchill Livingston, New York, 1988, pp. 81–100.
5. Blessing J, Anderson B: Analysis of clinical trials in gynecologic cancer—timing and interpretation. *Gynecol Oncol* 1986; 23:275.

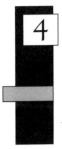

4

THE ROLE OF CHEMOTHERAPY IN GYNECOLOGIC CANCER

CHRISTINA S. CHU AND J. TATE THIGPEN

Knowledge about the use of chemotherapy in gynecologic cancers has expanded rapidly over the last two decades because of the effective use of large cooperative trials. Specific neoplasms for which there is at least some scientific basis for systemic therapy include celomic epithelial carcinoma of the ovary, endometrial carcinoma, carcinoma of the cervix, uterine sarcomas, gestational trophoblastic disease, and germ cell cancers of the ovary.

▓▓▓▓ *Epithelial Carcinoma of the Ovary*

Epithelial carcinomas of the ovary constitute the second most common cancer of the female genital tract (90% of the projected 25,400 new cases of cancer of the ovary in 2003) and the most common cause of death due to gynecologic cancer (90% of the projected 14,300 deaths due to cancer of the ovary in 2003). The neoplasm arises from the celomic epithelium, which invests the ovary during development and also lines the entire peritoneal cavity; hence, the disease process develops intraabdominally and spreads initially by seeding throughout the peritoneum. The most important prognostic factor is the extent of disease at the time of diagnosis as expressed in the International Federation of Gynecology and Obstetrics (FIGO) staging system (Table 4.1). Seventy-five percent of patients present with stage III or IV

Chemotherapy of Gynecologic Cancers: Society of Gynecologic Oncologists Handbook 2e, edited by Stephen C. Rubin, MD, Lippincott Williams & Wilkins, Philadelphia © 2004.

■ Table 4.1
FIGO Staging System for Carcinoma of the Ovary

Stage		Description
I		Growth limited to the ovaries
	A	One ovary; no ascites; capsule intact; no tumor on external surface
	B	Two ovaries; no ascites; capsule intact; no tumor on external surface
	C	One or both ovaries with surface tumor, ruptured capsule, or ascites or peritoneal washings with malignant cells
II		Pelvic extension
	A	Involvement of uterus and/or tubes
	B	Involvement of other pelvic tissues
	C	IIA or IIB with factors as in IC
III		Peritoneal implants outside pelvis and/or positive retroperitoneal or inguinal nodes
	A	Grossly limited to true pelvis; negative nodes; microscopic seeding of abdominal peritoneum
	B	Implants of abdominal peritoneum ≤2 cm; nodes negative
	C	Abdominal implants >2 cm and/or positive retroperitoneal or inguinal nodes
IV		Distant metastases

(advanced) disease because of the lack of an effective method of early diagnosis. Stage III is the most common stage at presentation (50% of all cases) as a consequence of the propensity of the tumor to spread by intraperitoneal dissemination.

These facts have an important impact on the role of chemotherapy. First, the intraabdominal nature of the disease necessitates that an exploratory laparotomy be done to accurately stage the patient before any decision is made regarding chemotherapy. Second, because the disease usually presents at an advanced stage, systemic therapy is the mainstay of management. Third, the confinement of the bulk of disease to the peritoneal cavity renders the disease amenable to surgical cytoreduction, which in turn enhances the response rate to chemotherapy and the resultant survival in those patients whose residual disease does not include any nodule larger than 2 cm in diameter and particularly in those in whom all gross disease can be resected.

■■■ Chemotherapy in Advanced Disease

After completion of surgical cytoreduction, the 75% of patients who have advanced (stage III or IV) disease will require chemotherapy. Approximately 40% of these advanced disease patients will have small-volume residual disease (no nodule larger than 2 cm) at the conclusion of surgery.

ACTIVE DRUGS

A number of cytotoxic drugs are active against carcinoma of the ovary. Generally regarded as the most active and most important are the platinum compounds, cisplatin and carboplatin. Based on seven randomized trials of cisplatin-versus carboplatin-based regimens, these two agents appear to be therapeutically equivalent. Although carboplatin produces more myelosuppression than cisplatin, it causes less nephrotoxicity and neurotoxicity and appears to have an advantage in terms of therapeutic index.

The taxanes appear to be the second most important group of agents. Both paclitaxel and docetaxel have been used in clinical trials of ovarian carcinoma. Although docetaxel causes more myelosuppression, paclitaxel appears to cause more peripheral neuropathy. Both agents are clearly active, and clinical resistance to one agent does not necessarily preclude response to the other.

Other agents active against ovarian carcinoma include the anthracyclines (doxorubicin and liposomal doxorubicin), gemcitabine, hexamethylmelamine, topotecan, vinorelbine, etoposide, 5-fluorouracil, methotrexate, mitomycin C, progestins, tamoxifen, and the interferons. Alkylating agents such as melphalan, cyclophosphamide, and ifosfamide also have activity against ovarian carcinoma.

REGIMEN OF CHOICE

Over the last two decades, major clinical trials have provided a solid basis for the selection of a drug regimen. The combination of a platinum and a taxane should be considered the standard of care for first-line treatment of advanced disease. Both GOG 111 and OV10 (the European-Canadian Intergroup Trial) were large phase 3 randomized trials that demonstrated improvements in both time to progression and median survival for patients receiving cisplatin/paclitaxel versus cisplatin/cyclophosphamide. Although the ICON3 study showed no difference in overall survival for patients treated with carboplatin alone compared to those receiving carboplatin/paclitaxel, this study used less strict eligibility criteria, treated a heterogenous population of patients, and should not be considered the basis for deferring treatment with a taxane. The GOG is currently conducting a large phase 3 randomized trial of first-line therapy comparing carboplatin/paclitaxel to four other arms using carboplatin/paclitaxel plus topotecan, gemcitabine, or liposomal doxorubicin. Until the results of this trial are complete, platinum/taxane combination regimens that have been shown to yield a statistically superior response rate, progression-free survival, and overall survival and should be regarded as the chemotherapy regimen of choice for patients with newly diagnosed advanced disease.

Consolidation therapy is controversial. A Southwest Oncology Group and GOG trial comparing 12 versus 3 months of single-agent paclitaxel for clinical complete responders showed a statistically significant improvement in progression-free survival for patients randomized to receive 12 cycles of therapy (28 months vs. 21 months). However, because results met criteria for early termination, the study was discontinued before achieving full accrual goals. Of note, evaluation of survival is not possible because too few events had occurred at the time of the study was stopped; and extensive cross-over after study closure makes further survival data unreliable for purposes of comparison. While consolidation with monthly paclitaxel may be a reasonable option, confirmation is needed before this approach can be declared the standard of care. For now, the issue should be discussed thoroughly with each patient; and the patient should participate in the decision as to whether to use maintenance paclitaxel.

Intraperitoneal chemotherapy has also been studied. GOG 104 randomized patients with optimal stage III disease to receive either intravenous cyclophosphamide/cisplatin or intravenous cyclophosphamide and intraperitoneal cisplatin. Patients receiving intraperitoneal cisplatin had a higher pathologic complete response rate (25% vs. 20%) as well as a longer median survival (49 months vs. 41 months). More recently, early results from GOG 172 have confirmed a modest improvement in recurrence risk for optimal stage III patients randomized to receive intravenous paclitaxel followed by intraperitoneal cisplatin/paclitaxel as compared to intravenous paclitaxel/cisplatin, though patients receiving intraperitoneal therapy had significantly increased rates of hematologic, gastrointestinal, renal, neurologic, infectious, metabolic, and pain toxicity. If the use of intraperitoneal therapy is to be considered, toxicity should be thoroughly discussed with the patient.

■■■■ Chemotherapy in Limited Disease

Patients with limited (stage I or II) disease should be classified as either high risk or low risk for recurrence based on the pathological features of the disease. Those considered at low risk should display all of the following characteristics: grade 1 or 2 disease, no tumor excrescences on the surface of the ovary (intracystic disease), no ascites, negative peritoneal cytology, and no extraovarian spread. Patients should be classified as high risk if any one of the following is present: grade 3 disease, tumor excrescences on the surface of the ovary (extracystic disease), ascites, positive peritoneal cytology, or extraovarian spread.

For the low-risk patients, total abdominal hysterectomy, bilateral salpingo-oophorectomy, omentectomy, and careful exploration of the abdomen yield a 5-year survival rate that exceeds 90%. Surgery alone is therefore the treatment of choice. For the high-risk patients, however, surgery alone produces a 5-year survival rate of no more than 60%; hence, the use of adjuvant therapy is appropriate. GOG 157 randomized patients with stage IA grade 3, stage IB grade 3, stage IC, and completely resected stage II disease to receive either 3 or 6 courses of carboplatin/paclitaxel. Preliminary results show an estimated probability of recurrence within 5 years of 27% versus 19%, respectively. Though no statistically significant difference in the rate of recurrence was noted, hematologic and neurotoxicity were significantly greater in patients receiving six cycles. Three cycles of platinum/taxane chemotherapy should be regarded as the current treatment of choice for high-risk patients with early stage disease.

Chemotherapy in Recurrent Disease

The management of recurrent ovarian carcinoma is dictated by the results of therapy at the time of initial diagnosis. Patients who responded to initial platinum-based therapy and experienced a treatment-free interval of 6 months or more are considered to be clinically platinum sensitive. Those who progress while on initial platinum-based therapy, whose best response to initial therapy is stable disease, or who relapse after initial response within 6 months of completion of platinum-based therapy are considered to be clinically platinum resistant.

Patients who are classified as clinically sensitive should receive platinum-based combination chemotherapy (paclitaxel followed by cisplatin). Response rates as high as 60% have been reported in this situation. As long as the patient responds and experiences at least a 6-month treatment-free interval after each successive application of platinum-based chemotherapy, treatment upon relapse should be repeat platinum-based chemotherapy. The ICON4 trial indicated that patients with recurrence longer than 6 months after completion of last therapy may benefit from platinum plus paclitaxel as opposed to other platinum-based regimens, with improvements in survival and progression-free survival, though fewer than 50% of patients studied had received prior treatment with a taxane. The benefit was more pronounced in those patients relapsing greater than 12 months from prior treatment. For those patients who are clinically resistant, choice of drugs should focus on those with demonstrated activity against taxane-platinum resistant disease: alternative taxane of taxane schedule, liposomal doxorubicin, topotecan, gemcitabine, and oral etoposide.

▬▬ Summary

For patients with advanced disease (Table 4.2), an aggressive attempt at surgical cytoreduction should be followed by combination chemotherapy: 175 mg/m^2 paclitaxel over 3 hours followed by carboplatin AUC 6 to 7.5 repeated every 3 weeks for six to eight cycles. In those patients who cannot take carboplatin, 75 mg/m^2 cisplatin administered at a rate of 1 mg/min may be substituted and the paclitaxel dose decreased to 135 mg/m^2 over 24 hours. Docetaxel may also be substituted for paclitaxel in cases where peripheral neuropathy is of particular concern. In large-vol-

▬▬ Table 4.2
Recommendations for the Management of Epithelial Carcinoma of the Ovary

Disease Status	Recommendation
Advanced Disease	Aggressive attempt at surgical cytoreduction followed by platinum/taxane
Limited Disease	
Low risk	Total abdominal hysterectomy, bilateral salpingooophorectomy, and omentectomy followed by observation
High risk	Total abdominal hysterectomy, bilateral salpingooophorectomy, and omentectomy followed by adjuvant platinum/taxane
Recurrent Disease	
Platinum-sensitive	Platinum-based single agent or combination chemotherapy (taxane/platinum)
Platinum-resistant	Treatment with potentially non-cross-resistant agents (taxane, liposomal doxorubicin, topotecan, gemcitabine, and oral etoposide)

ume disease, this should yield a response rate of 77%, a clinical complete response rate of 54%, a median progression-free survival of 18 months, and a median survival exceeding 36 months. Long-term survival should exceed 20%. In small-volume disease, these results should be proportionately better.

For patients with limited disease, no adjuvant chemotherapy is indicated for those deemed to be at low risk with an expected 5-year survival exceeding 90%. Those at high risk have an expected 5-year survival no better than 60% and should receive adjuvant platinum/taxane chemotherapy with an expected improvement to a 5-year survival of 80%.

Recurrent disease should be treated with platinum-based chemotherapy if the disease exhibits characteristics associated with platinum sensitivity. A response rate as high as 60% should be expected. For those patients with platinum-resistant disease, other drugs to be considered in those who have progressed on a platinum plus paclitaxel regimen include taxanes, liposomal doxorubicin, topotecan, gemcitabine, and oral etoposide.

Several other therapeutic options, such as high-dose chemotherapy supported by autologous bone marrow transplantation and abdominopelvic radiation, have been widely discussed. No evidence supports the use of these approaches outside of a clinical trial.

Endometrial Carcinoma

Endometrial carcinoma is the most common invasive malignancy of the female genital tract, with an expected 40,100 new cases in the United States in 2003. Because the disease produces vaginal bleeding early in its course, diagnosis at a limited stage is the rule; hence, only 6,800 deaths are projected to occur in 2003. The most important prognostic factor is the extent of disease at the time of diagnosis as expressed in the FIGO staging system (Table 4.3). Stage I disease (confined to the corpus) accounts for 75% of all

■■■ Table 4.3
FIGO Staging System for Endometrial Carcinoma

Stage	Description
IA G123	Tumor limited to the endometrium
IB G123	Invasion to less than half of myometrium
IC G123	Invasion to more than half of myometrium
IIA G123	Endocervical glandular involvement only
IIB G123	Cervical stromal invasion
IIIA G123	Tumor invades serosa or adnexae or positive peritoneal cytology
IIIB G123	Vaginal metastases
IIIC G123	Metastases to pelvic or para-aortic lymph nodes
IVA G123	Tumor invasion of bladder and/or bowel mucosa
IVB	Distant metastases including intra-abdominal and/or inguinal lymph nodes

cases and stage II (involvement of the cervix) accounts for an additional 13%. The 5-year survival rate for all patients is 66%. The role of chemotherapy for the treatment of patients with endometrial cancer is under active investigation in a number of phase 2 randomized trials. Active systemic agents include doxorubicin, the platinum compounds, fluorouracil, cyclophosphamide, ifosfamide, and paclitaxel. Each yields a single-agent response rate in excess of 20%. Of note, paclitaxel has been shown to have response rates of 27% to 38% in the salvage setting. Patients with advanced or recurrent disease not amenable to surgery or radiation should receive chemotherapy. A initial randomized trial showed a clear advantage for combination chemotherapy consisting of 60 mg/m^2 doxorubicin plus 50 mg/m^2 cisplatin every 3 weeks as compared to single-agent doxorubicin. Because of phase 2 trials documenting response rates of 27% to 38% with the use of paclitaxel in the salvage setting, the drug has been studied in various combinations with cisplatin and doxorubicin. Preliminary results have shown no difference in response rates between cisplatin/doxorubicin and paclitaxel/doxorubicin, but early results from GOG 177 have demonstrated improved response rate and progression-free and overall survival for the three-drug combination of doxorubicin/cisplatin/paclitaxel compared to doxorubicin/cisplatin, though more toxicity was incurred. The combination of paclitaxel/carboplatin has also been studied in the phase 2 setting, with response rates of 50% to 78% and associated minimal toxicity. Because of these promising results, the GOG is currently conducting a phase 3 trial randomizing patients to doxorubicin/cisplatin/ paclitaxel or carboplatin/paclitaxel.

Hormonal therapies have also shown limited efficacy in patients with endometrial cancer. Candidates for progestins or tamoxifen include those with disease positive for estrogen and progesterone receptors or, in the absence of receptor levels, those with other than grade 3 disease, which has only a 25% probability of being receptor positive. If hormonal therapy is to be used, progestins are the usual choice, with an expected response rate of 20%. Objective evidence supports the daily use of 200 mg medroxyprogesterone acetate orally or 160 mg megestrol acetate orally; a randomized trial showed no advantage to higher doses.

Although high-risk categories of patients can be identified among those with stage I-III disease, no current evidence defines a role for systemic therapy in these patients except in those patients with stage III-IVA disease. GOG Protocol 122 compared surgery followed by abdomino-pelvic radiation to surgery followed by doxorubicin/cisplatin and showed superior progression-free and overall survival for those patients treated with surgery followed by chemotherapy. Currently, the GOG is accruing patients to protocol 184, which is a randomized study of tumor volume directed radiation followed by doxorubicin/cisplatin or doxorubicin/cisplatin/paclitaxel in patients with surgical stage III disease.

Treatment recommendations for the use of chemotherapy are summarized in Table 4.4. In brief, patients with disseminated or recurrent disease should receive systemic therapy. The combination of doxorubicin/cisplatin/paclitaxel provides an improvement in response rate and progression-free

▆▆ Table 4.4

Recommendations for the Use of Systemic Therapy in Endometrial Carcinoma

Patient Characteristics	Recommendations
Advanced or recurrent disease	Chemotherapy (cisplatin/doxorubicin/ paclitaxel)
Advanced or recurrent receptor-positive and/or grade 1 or 2	Hormonal therapy (oral progestins or megestrol acetate)
Stage III-IVA	Surgery followed by chemotherapy

and overall survival compared with doxorubicin/cisplatin. Hormonal therapy with progestins is appropriate for those with disease features suggesting hormonal responsiveness. Chemotherapy for patients with stage III-IVA disease should be considered following surgery.

▆▆▆ *Carcinoma of the Uterine Cervix*

Carcinoma of the uterine cervix remains a common disease, although the majority of cases are diagnosed before invasion, with cure the expected result, at least in the United States. In 2003, a projected 12,200 invasive cases with 4,100 deaths are expected, a marked reduction from the almost 60,000 deaths from this disease in 1950. The majority of cases are squamous carcinomas (80%–85%); hence, most of the data on management apply most reliably to this histologic type. The approach to other histologies is based on the assumption that histology does not alter therapeutic choices, at least in the case of systemic therapy. For invasive cases, management is dictated by the extent of disease at diagnosis as expressed in the FIGO staging system (Table 4.5). Chemotherapy has a defined role in two situations: the management of advanced (stage IVB) or recurrent disease as the primary therapy, and the management of locoregionally advanced (stage IIB, III, or IVA) disease in conjunction with radiation.

▬▬ Table 4.5
FIGO Staging System for Carcinoma of the Cervix

Stage	Description
Stage I	The carcinoma is strictly confined to the cervix
IA	Invasive cancer identified only microscopically. All gross lesions even with superficial invasion are stage IB cancers
	Invasion is limited to measured stromal invasion with maximum depth of 5.0 mm and no wider than 7.0 mm*
IA1	Measured invasion of stroma no greater than 3.0 mm in depth and no wider than 7.0 mm
IA2	Measured invasion of stroma greater than 3 mm and no greater than 5 mm and no wider than 7 mm
IB	Clinical lesions confined to the cervix or preclinical lesions greater than stage IA
IB1	Clinical lesions no greater than 4.0 cm in size
IB2	Clinical lesions greater than 4.0 cm in size
Stage II	Vaginal or parametrial extension
IIA	Extension to the upper two-thirds of vagina
IIB	Extension to parametria, but not to pelvic sidewall
Stage III	Pelvic sidewall extension, lower vaginal involvement, or hydronephrosis
IIIA	Extension to the lower one-third of vagina
IIIB	Extension to pelvic sidewall or hydronephrosis
Stage IV	Mucosal involvement of bladder or rectum, or distant disease
IVA	Mucosal involvement of bladder or rectum
IVB	Involvement of distant organs

* The depth of invasion should not be more than 5 mm taken from the base of the epithelium, either surface or glandular, from which it originates. Vascular space involvement, either venous or lymphatic, should not alter the staging.

▬▬ Advanced or Recurrent Disease

In patients with advanced or recurrent disease, a number of cytotoxic drugs have minimal to moderate activity (response rates of 10%–15%), but several agents or groups of agents have shown consistent activity in the range of response rates of better than 15%. The most intensely studied agent is cisplatin, which demonstrated a response rate of 23% among 815 patients studied by the GOG in trials of single-agent cisplatin. Activity does not appear to depend on dose and schedule as long as at least 50 mg/m^2 is used every 3 weeks. In the absence of major antiemetics (metoclopramide, ondansetron, and granisetron), infusion over 24 hours rather than at 1 mg/min yields less nausea and vomiting. Carboplatin appears to have a slightly lower response rate in the range of 15% to 20%, although this agent has never been directly compared to cisplatin in a phase III trial in cervix carcinoma.

Other active agents used as monotherapy include ifosfamide, vinorelbine, paclitaxel, topotecan, and irinotecan. Ifosfamide, in several smaller trials, produced responses in up to 33% of patients not previously exposed to chemotherapy. Phase 2 trials of vinorelbine have reported response rates of 18% in patients with prior radiation, and 45% when used as neoadjuvant therapy. Paclitaxel, topotecan, and irinotecan have all shown responses of approximately 17% to 20% among patients who have been treated with radiation.

It is important to note that responses to single-agent therapy usually result in responses of relatively brief duration, except for the 5% to 10% who achieve a complete response. Although such therapy should be considered as an option and so presented to the patient, expectations of benefit must be tempered.

A few large randomized trials of combination chemotherapy versus single agents have been conducted. GOG Protocol 110 randomized patients with advanced or recurrent disease to receive cisplatin alone, cisplatin/dibromodulcitol, or cisplatin/ifosfamide. Response rates were 19%, 22%, and 33%, respectively. No significant difference was noted in the response rates between cisplatin alone and cisplatin/dibromodulcitol. However, the combination of cisplatin/ifosfamide produced a significantly improved response rate and progression-free survival but at the cost of increased hematologic, renal, and neurologic toxicity. No difference in overall survival was noted. GOG 169 randomized patients with stage IVB, recurrent, or persistent disease to receive either cisplatin alone or cisplatin/paclitaxel. The majority of patients had received radiation therapy. Preliminary results document significantly improved response rate (19% vs. 36%, respectively) and progression free-survival (2.8 months vs. 4.8 months, respectively). No difference was noted in median survival. Although the combination incurred more frequent neutropenia and anemia, no significant differences were noted in patient-reported quality of life.

Randomized trials comparing various chemotherapeutic combinations have not shown a clear benefit. GOG 149 compared cisplatin and ifosfamide with or without bleomycin for the treatment of advanced, recurrent, or persistent disease showed no difference in response, progression-free interval, survival, or toxicity. Currently, the GOG has completed a comparison of topotecan/cisplatin versus cisplatin alone and is conducting a phase 3 randomized trial of cisplatin plus either paclitaxel, or vinorelbine. Until additional results are available, the current data suggest that cisplatin/paclitaxel or cisplatin/ifosfamide may offer patients higher response rate and superior progression-free survival, though with increased toxicity.

▰▰▰▰ Locoregionally Advanced Disease

The role of chemotherapy in the treatment of cervical cancer has changed dramatically in the last several years, with the concurrent use of platinum-based therapy with radiation becoming the standard of care for treatment of locally advanced cervical cancer (IIB-IVA). Five randomized phase 3 trials were published in 1999 and 2000 (Table 4.6). Although these trials treated different groups of patients with differing regimens of chemotherapy and radiation, all showed statistically significant overall survival advantage for concurrent platinum-based chemotherapy. Survival was improved in patients with locally advanced cervical cancer (stages IB-IVA), as well as those with stage I-IIA disease with poor prognostic factors such

Table 4.6
Summary of Chemoradiation Trials for Cervical Cancer

Protocol	Eligible Patients	Treatment Arms	3-Year Survival (%)
GOG 85 (SWOG 8695)	Stages IIB-IVA Negative para-aortic nodes No intraperitoneal disease	I: pelvic EBRT, brachytherapy 5-FU/cisplatin II: pelvic EBRT, brachytherapy hydroxyurea	67 57
RTOG 9001	Stages IIB-IVA, or Stage IB and IA with positive pelvic nodes or tumor > 5cm	I: pelvic EBRT, brachytherapy 5-FU/cisplatin II: extended-field EBRT, brachytherapy	75 63
GOG 120	Stages IIB-IVA Negative para-aortic nodes No intraperitoneal disease	I: pelvic EBRT, brachytherapy weekly cisplatin II: pelvic EBRT, brachytherapy 5-FU/cisplatin/hydroxyurea III: pelvic EBRT, brachytherapy hydroxyurea	65 65 47
SWOG 8797 (GOG 109, RTOG 9112)	Stages IA2, IB, IIA with positive pelvic nodes, positive parametria, or positive surgical margins Negative para-aortic nodes	I: pelvic EBRT, brachytherapy 5-FU/cisplatin II: pelvic EBRT	87 77
GOG 123	Stage IB2 Negative pelvic and para-aortic nodes	I: pelvic EBRT, brachytherapy weekly cisplatin extrafascial hysterectomy II: pelvic EBRT, brachytherapy extrafascial hysterectomy	83 74 (median follow-up 35.7 mo)

GOG, Gynecologic Oncology Group; SWOG, Southwest Oncology Group; RTOG, Radiation Therapy Oncology Group; EBRT, external beam radiation therapy.

■ Table 4.7
Recommendations for the Use of Chemotherapy in Carcinoma of the Cervix

Patient Characteristics	Recommendations
Stage IVB or recurrent disease	Chemotherapy (combination of cisplatin plus ifosfamide or cisplatin plus paclitaxel)
Stages IIB, III, IVA	Radiotherapy with concomitant chemotherapy (cisplatin/5-fluorouracil or weekly cisplatin)

as positive surgical margins, parametria, or pelvic nodes. Chemoradiation appears to decrease the risk of death by approximately 30% to 50%. Though the single best chemotherapy regimen has not been defined, both weekly cisplatin alone and the combination of cisplatin/fluorouracil both appear effective with acceptable toxicity.

■ Summary

Chemotherapy should be considered in two situations: advanced or recurrent disease as the primary treatment, and locoregionally advanced disease in combination with radiotherapy (Table 4.7). In advanced or recurrent disease, combination therapy with cisplatin/paclitaxel or cisplatin/ifosfamide may result in a longer progression-free survival and a higher response rate than cisplatin alone, though overall survival has not shown to be significantly increased. In locoregionally advanced disease, concurrent cisplatin/fluorouracil or weekly cisplatin should be given concurrently with radiation.

■ *Uterine Sarcomas*

Uterine sarcomas account for fewer than 5% of cancers of the corpus of the uterus. In the United States, this translates into approximately 1,000 cases per year. Although multiple histologic types are seen, the GOG experience observes that 60% will be malignant mixed mullerian tumors, 30%

▬ Table 4.8
Staging Criteria for Uterine Sarcomas (modified from FIGO staging of endometrial cancer)

Stage	Description
I	Sarcoma confined to the uterine corpus
II	Sarcoma confined to corpus and cervix
III	Sarcoma confined to pelvis
IV	Extrapelvic sarcoma

leiomyosarcomas, and 10% other types including endometrial stromal sarcomas. Management is dictated by the modified FIGO staging criteria (Table 4.8). The defined role of chemotherapy is confined to the treatment of patients with disseminated or recurrent disease. Choice of regimen is determined by the histology, with most available information provided by GOG trials.

For patients with advanced or recurrent malignant mixed mullerian tumors, three clearly active agents have been identified: ifosfamide (32% response rate), cisplatin (19% response rate), and paclitaxel (18% response rate). Other agents studied (including doxorubicin) have yielded response rates of less than 10%. The combination of ifosfamide/cisplatin may provide a small increase in progression-free survival, but no improvement in overall survival has been noted. Currently, the combination of ifosfamide/paclitaxel versus ifosfamide alone is being studied by the GOG.

For patients with advanced or recurrent leiomyosarcomas, only one agent has yielded better than a 15% response rate: doxorubicin (25%). No advantage has been shown for combinations of doxorubicin with either DTIC or ifosfamide, two drugs popular for combination regimens with doxorubicin. Current research efforts are focusing on the identification of additional active agents.

No studies to date have shown efficacy for chemotherapy in the adjuvant setting even though stage I cases have recurrence rates as high as 50%. The GOG is currently con-

▬▬ Table 4.9
Recommendations for the Use of Chemotherapy in Advanced
or Recurrent Uterine Sarcomas

Histology	Recommendation
Mixed mesodermal sarcoma	Chemotherapy (single-agent ifosfamide or a combination of ifosfamide/cisplatin)
Leiomyosarcoma	Chemotherapy (single-agent doxorubicin)
Other histologies	Data inconclusive

ducting a study of whole-abdominal radiotherapy versus ifosfamide/cisplatin for optimally debulked stage I-IV.

The recommendations for the use of chemotherapy in uterine sarcomas are summarized in Table 4.9.

▬▬ Ovarian Germ Cell Cancers

Ovarian germ cell cancers account for only 5% of all ovarian cancers. From the standpoint of chemotherapy, histology is divided into the dysgerminomas and the nondysgerminomas. The role of systemic therapy is clearer for the nondysgerminomas than for the dysgerminomas; hence, the following section will deal primarily with nondysgerminomas, but the recommendations are probably applicable to dysgerminomas. Treatment is dictated by the extent of disease (FIGO staging system as described in Table 4.1) and the completeness of surgical resection. For purposes of therapeutic decision making, patients will be divided into those with completely resected and those with incompletely resected tumors.

For patients with stage IV or incompletely resected neoplasms, systemic therapy is the treatment of choice. The optimal regimen appears to be a combination of bleomycin plus etoposide plus cisplatin (BEP): 20 U/m^2 bleomycin i.v. (maximum, 30 U) weekly for 12 doses, 100 mg/m^2 etoposide i.v. daily for 5 days every 3 weeks for four cycles, and 20 mg/m^2 cisplatin i.v. daily for 5 days every 3 weeks for four cycles. Response rates should exceed 90%, complete responses 70%. More than 50% of patients will be long-term survivors and possible cures.

For patients with completely resected disease, the need for adjuvant therapy is determined to some extent by histology. For patients with immature teratomas grade 1, no further treatment appears indicated. Patients with completely staged IA dysgerminomas may also be observed, though 20% may recur; these patients may be successfully treated at the time of recurrence. For all others, adjuvant treatment with BEP as described above for three cycles should be considered for patients with completely resected disease, and four cycles for those with incompletely resected disease. With BEP, relapse rates are less than 5%, whereas no adjuvant treatment is associated with relapse rates ranging from 40% to 80%.

For patients unable to take BEP, enhanced results are reported with a combination of vincristine, actinomycin D, and cyclophosphamide, but these results are clearly inferior to those achieved with BEP.

The recommendations for the use of chemotherapy in patients with germ cell cancers of the ovary are summarized in Table 4.10.

■■■■ Table 4.10
Recommendations for the Use of Chemotherapy in Germ Cell Cancers of the Ovary

Patient Characteristics	Recommendations
Incompletely resected	Four cycles of BEP*
Completely resected	Three cycles of BEP* or, if BEP cannot be given, six cycles of VAC**
Stage IA1 immature teratoma	Observation
Stage IA dysgerminoma	Observation

 * BEP: Bleomycin 20 units/m^2 IV (max 30 units) weekly
   Etoposide 100 mg/m^2 IV daily × 5 q 3 weeks
   Cisplatin 20 mg/m^2 IV daily × 5 q 3 weeks
 ** VAC: Vincristine 1.5 mg/m^2 IV (max 2 mg) q 2 weeks
   Actinomycin D 350 μg/m^2 IV daily × 5 days q 4 weeks
   Cyclophosphamide 150 mg/m^2 IV daily × 5 days q 4 weeks

▪▪▪▪ *Gestational Trophoblastic Disease*

Gestational trophoblastic disease arising in the placenta includes a spectrum of neoplastic processes including molar pregnancy, invasive mole, and choriocarcinoma. Although uncommon, the disease process is important because it is amenable to cure even in advanced stages of spread. Diagnosis rests on the demonstration of a rising or plateauing human chorionic gonadotropin (HCG) level after evacuation of a hydatidiform mole, a histologic diagnosis of invasive mole or choriocarcinoma, or a persistent elevation of HCG levels with or without objective evidence of metastases following a pregnancy. Approximately 50% of all cases follow a hydatidiform mole, 25% an abortion, and 25% a normal pregnancy.

Regarding the use of chemotherapy, patients should be separated into three groups: nonmetastatic disease, metastatic disease at low risk, and metastatic disease at high risk. Assignment to a group requires that the patient be assessed for extent of disease as follows: the measurement of the β-subunit of HCG and examination of the likely sites of spread (abdomen and pelvis, lungs, and brain). Assignment is based on a staging system developed by the International Society for the Study of Trophoblastic Neoplasms. Stage I patients (nonmetastatic disease) have disease confined to the uterus (Table 4.11). Assignment of patients to the other two groups depends on additional variables. The National Cancer Institute (NCI) recognizes several high-risk factors including pretreatment HCG level greater than 100,000 IU/24 hours (urine) or 40,000 IU/mL (serum), time from antecedent event to treatment longer than 4 months, antecedent term pregnancy, metastases to sites other than lungs and vagina, prior unsuccessful chemotherapy, and antecedent term gestation. The World Health Organization (WHO) uses a prognostic scoring system based on age, antecedent pregnancy, interval to diagnosis, maternal/paternal blood type, size of primary tumor, size of metastatic lesions, number of metastases, and prior chemotherapy. The pres-

▪▪ Table 4.11

FIGO Staging System for Gestational Trophoblastic Tumors

Stage	Description
I	Disease confined to the uterus
IA	Disease confined to the uterus, with no risk factor
IB	Disease confined to the uterus, with one risk factor
IC	Disease confined to the uterus, with two risk factors
II	Disease extending outside uterus but limited to genital structures
IIA	Disease extending outside uterus but limited to genital structures, with no risk factor
IIB	Disease extending outside uterus but limited to genital structures, with one risk factor
IIC	Disease extending outside uterus but limited to genital structures
III	Disease extending to lungs with or without known genital tract involvement
IIIA	Disease extending to lungs with or without known genital tract involvement, with no risk factor
IIIB	Disease extending to lungs with or without known genital tract involvement, with one risk factor
IIIC	Disease extending to lungs with or without known genital tract involvement, with two risk factors
IV	All other metastatic sites
IVA	All other metastatic sites, with no risk factor
IVB	All other metastatic sites, with one risk factor
IVC	All other metastatic sites, with two risk factors

Risk factors affecting staging include: (1) hCG>100,000 U/l and (2) duration of disease > 6 months from termination of antecedent pregnancy.

ence of one or more NCI poor prognostic factors or a WHO score of 8 or higher classifies a patient as high risk.

For patients with nonmetastatic gestational trophoblastic disease, single-agent chemotherapy with either actinomycin D or methotrexate is the standard of care. Hysterectomy may be performed if the patient has completed childbearing. If actinomycin D is used, two schedules are acceptable: 10 to 13 μg/kg daily for 5 days or 1.25 mg/m^2 once every 2 weeks. If methotrexate is chosen, three schedules are equivalent: 0.4 mg/kg daily for 5 days every 2 weeks; 1 mg/kg on days 1, 3, 5, 7, followed by leucovorin 0.1 mg/kg on days 2, 4, 6, 8, every 15 to 18 days; and methotrexate 30 to 50 mg/m^2 i.m. weekly. Therapy is generally continued until negative HCG measurements are obtained. Cure is expected in 85% to 90% of patients with the initial regimen. Should HCG levels plateau or rise after two courses or toxicity preclude adequate doses of therapy, treatment should be changed to the alternative single agent, MAC (methotrexate, actinomycin D, and cyclophosphamide or chlorambucil) combination therapy, and/or hysterectomy.

For patients with low-risk metastatic disease, single-agent chemotherapy as described for nonmetastatic disease should be used, with greater than 80% of patients achieving complete remission. The need to change therapy is determined by a plateau or rise in the HCG level on two consecutive samples or the appearance of new sites of metastases. Nearly all patients in whom single-agent therapy fails may achieve remission with combination chemotherapy.

Whereas virtually all patients with low-risk metastatic disease will respond to single agents, only 20% of patients with high-risk metastatic disease respond when treated with single-agent therapy Although triple agent therapy with MAC has been used in the setting of high-risk disease, only about 50% of patient with a WHO score of 8 or higher will achieve complete remission. The EMA-CO regimen (etoposide, methotrexate, actinomycin D, cyclophosphamide, and vincristine) is the current treatment of choice for patients with high-risk metastatic disease, with reported cure rates ranging from 70% to 90%. More than 80% of those refractory to EMA-CO have been cured by additional treatment using etoposide and cisplatin instead of cyclophosphamide and vincristine (EMA-EP).

In summary, chemotherapy has a definite role in the management of patients with gestational trophoblastic disease. In those with nonmetastatic and low-risk metastatic disease, single-agent chemotherapy consisting of pulse-dose methotrexate or actinomycin D is recommended. Pa-

Table 4.12
Chemotherapy Regimens for Gestational Trophoblastic Disease

Patient Chacteristics	Regimen	Schedule and Doses	Regimen	Repeated
Non-metastatic or Low-risk metastatic disease	MTX, or	Methotrexate	1 mg/kg IM days 1, 3, 5, 7	Every 2 weeks
		Leucovorin	0.1 mg/kg IM days 2, 4, 6, 8	
	Act-D	Actinomycin D	10–13 mcg/kg IV daily for 5 days	Every 12 d
Refractory disease	MAC	Methotrexate	0.3 mg/kg IV × 5 days	Every 3 wks
		Actinomycin	8 mcg/kg IV × 5 days	
		Chlorambucil*	0.15 mg/kg IV × 5 days	
High-risk metastatic disease	EMA-CO	Etoposide	100 mg/m^2 IV days 1–2	Every 2 wks
		Actinomycin	0.5 mg IV push days 1–2	
		Methotrexate	100 mg/m^2 IV push, then 200 mg/m^2 IV over 12h day 1	
		Leucovorin	15 mg IM or PO q 12 h × 4 24h after MTX	
		Vincristine	1 mg/m^2 IV push day 8	
Refractory disease	EMA-EP	Cyclophosphamide	600 mg/m^2 IV push day 8	
		Etoposide **	100 mg/m2 IV push day 8	
		Cisplatin **	80 mg/m2 IV day 8	

* may substitute cyclophosphamide 3 mg/kg IV × 5 days
* may substitute cyclophosphamide 3 mg/kg IV × 5 days
** same as EMA-CO, except substitute etoposide/cisplatin for vincristine cyclophosphamide

tients in whom initial therapy fails may be treated with the alternate single-agent or with MAC combination therapy. Patients with high-risk metastatic disease require combination chemotherapy with EMA-CO (Table 4.12). Patients with disease refractory to EMA-CO may be treated with etoposide/cisplatin regimens.

Selected Reading

████ Epithelial Carcinoma of the Ovary

Kim RY, Omura GA, Alvarez RD: Advances in the treatment of gynecologic malignancies. Part 2: Cancers of the uterine corpus and ovary. *Oncology (Huntingt)* 2002; 16:1669–78.

International Collaborative Ovarian Neoplasm Group: Paclitaxel plus carboplatin versus standard chemotherapy with either single-agent carboplatin or cyclophosphamide, doxorubicin, and cisplatin in women with ovarian cancer: The ICON3 randomised trial. *Lancet* 2002; 360:505–15.

Parmar MK, Ledermann JA, Colombo N, du Bois A, Delaloye JF, Kristensen GB, Wheeler S, Swart AM, Qian W, Torri V, Floriani I, Jayson G, Lamont A, Trope C: Paclitaxel plus platinum-based chemotherapy versus conventional platinum-based chemotherapy in women with relapsed ovarian cancer: the ICON4/AGO-OVAR-2.2 trial. *Lancet* 2003;361: 2099–2106.

McGuire WP, Hoskins WJ, Brady MF, Kucera PR, Partridge EE, Look KY, Clarke-Pearson DL, Davidson M: Cyclophosphamide and cisplatin compared with paclitaxel and cisplatin in patients with stage III and stage IV ovarian cancer. *N Engl J Med* 1996; 334:1–6.

████ Endometrial Carcinoma

Kim RY, Omura GA, Alvarez RD: Advances in the treatment of gynecologic malignancies. Part 2: Cancers of the uterine corpus and ovary. *Oncology (Huntingt)* 2002;16:1669–78.

Irvin WP, Rice LW, Berkowitz RS: Advances in the management of endometrial adenocarcinoma. A review. *J Reprod Med* 2002; 47:173–89.

Randall M, Brunetto G, Muss H, et al: Whole abdominal radiotherapy versus combination doxorubicin-cisplatin chemotherapy in advanced endometrial carcinoma: a randomized phase III trial of the Gynecologic Oncology Group. Proc ASCO 22: 2, 2003 (abstr 3).

████ Carcinoma of the Cervix

Kim RY, Alvarez RD, Omura GA: Advances in the treatment of gynecologic malignancies. Part 1: Cancers of the cervix and vulva. *Oncology (Huntingt)* 2002; 16:1510–17.

Whitney CW, Sause W, Bundy BN, et al: Randomized comparison of fluorouracil plus cisplatin versus hydroxyurea as an adjunct to radiation therapy in stage IIB-IVA carcinoma of the cervix with negative para-aortic lymph nodes: A Gynecologic Oncology Group and Southwest Oncology Group study. *J Clin Oncol* 1999; 17:1339–48.

Morris M, Eifel PJ, Lu J, et al: Pelvic radiation with concurrent chemotherapy compared with pelvic and para-aortic radiation for high-risk cervical cancer. *N Engl J Med* 1999; 340: 1137–43.

Rose PG, Bundy BN, Watkins EB, et al: Concurrent cisplatin-based radiotherapy and chemotherapy for locally advanced cervical cancer. *N Engl J Med* 1999; 340:1144–53.

Keys HM, Bundy BN, Stehman FB, et al: Cisplatin, radiation, and adjuvant hysterectomy compared with radiation and adjuvant hysterectomy for bulky stage IB cervical carcinoma. *N Engl J Med* 1999; 340:1154–1161.

Peters WA, Liu PY, Barrett RJ, et al: Concurrent chemotherapy and pelvic radiation therapy compared with pelvic radiation therapy alone as adjuvant therapy after radical surgery in high-risk early-stage cancer of the cervix. *J Clin Oncol* 2000; 18:1606–1613.

▬ Other Neoplasms

Berkowitz RS, Goldstein DP: Gestational trophoblastic diseases. In WJ Hosking, CA Perez, RC Young (eds.), *Principles and Practice of Gynecologic Oncology,* 3rd edition. Lippincott Williams & Wilkins, Philadelphia, 2000, pp. 1117–1137.

Hurteau JA, Williams SJ: Ovarian germ cell tumors. In SC Rubin SC, GP Sutton (eds.), *Ovarian Cancer,* 2nd edition, Lippincott Williams & Wilkins, Philadelphia, 2001, pp. 371–382.

Lurain JR: Advances in management of high-risk gestational trophoblastic tumors. *J Reprod Med* 2002; 47:451–459.

Thigpen JT: Chemotherapy of cancers of the female genital tract. In MC Perry (ed.), *The Chemotherapy Source Book*, Williams and Wilkins, Baltimore, 1992, pp. 1039–1067.

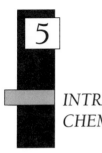

INTRAPERITONEAL CHEMOTHERAPY

MAURIE MARKMAN

Rationale and Pharmacology

The intraperitoneal (i.p.) administration of antineoplastic agents as treatment for gynecologic malignancies, specifically ovarian cancer or primary carcinoma of the peritoneum, is based on sound pharmacokinetic, anatomic, and physiological principles.

First, ovarian cancer remains principally confined to the peritoneal cavity in most individuals for the majority of its natural history. Second, the cancer usually grows on the surface of the peritoneal lining, rather than directly invading normal organs and tissue. Third, drug uptake from the peritoneal cavity is largely via the portal circulation. Thus, for drugs that are metabolized within the liver, the potential for a major pharmacokinetic advantage for peritoneal cavity exposure after i.p. drug delivery, compared with that of the systemic compartment, may exist. Even for agents that are not inactivated within the liver there may be a significant increase in tumor–drug interactions within the peritoneal cavity associated with i.p. drug administration.

There are a number of antineoplastic agents with known activity in ovarian cancer that may be considered for potential clinical utility in this setting. Of considerable interest are agents whose cytotoxicity, at least in experimental systems, exhibits steep dose–response curves, suggesting that, at the concentrations achievable, greater tumor cell

Chemotherapy of Gynecologic Cancers: Society of Gynecologic Oncologists Handbook 2e, edited by Stephen C. Rubin, MD, Lippincott Williams & Wilkins, Philadelphia © 2004.

████ Table 5.1.
Pharmacokinetic Advantage Associated With I.P. Delivery of Selected Drugs Active in Ovarian Cancer

	Ratio of Peritoneal Cavity/Plasma	
Agent	**Peak Levels**	**AUC***
Cisplatin	20	12
Carboplatin	—	18
Mitoxantrone	—	1,400
Doxorubicin	474	—
Mitomycin-C	71	—
Paclitaxel	1,000	1,000
Alpha-interferon	100	—

* Area under the concentration versus time curve.

kill may be observed within the peritoneal cavity after regional drug delivery.

Phase 1 clinical trials have demonstrated that for a number of agents with known activity in ovarian cancer there is a major pharmacokinetic advantage associated with i.p. drug delivery (Table 5.1). It is important to note that a major factor determining patient populations where i.p. delivery of antineoplastic agents may be a rational therapeutic option is the very limited ability of the drug to penetrate directly into tumor or normal tissue. This point will be highlighted in the discussion of clinical trials of i.p. cisplatin (see Efficacy).

████ Techniques

████ Access to the Peritoneal Cavity

Intraperitoneal delivery of cytotoxic agents can be accomplished either through a device placed at the time of each treatment (e.g., percutaneous paracentesis catheter or larger-bore catheter placed under laparoscopic control), or via a semipermanent indwelling catheter system (e.g., external Tenckhoff-type or subcutaneous port system attached to a catheter).

There are several advantages of placing a catheter with each treatment. The patient does not have to have a device in the abdominal cavity when she is not being treated, there is a lower chance of infection in the absence of a semipermanent indwelling catheter device, and the risk of slow erosion of the catheter into the bowel is eliminated. Disadvantages of this approach include the time, effort, and cost required for each treatment and the risk of acute bowel perforation, unless each insertion is done under direct visualization.

The advantages of semipermanent systems include the ease of administration (treatment can be delivered by the treating nurse) and reduced risk of complications of catheter insertion. Although there is a potentially higher risk of infection when catheters are left in the abdominal cavity for extended periods, this risk can be minimized by employing subcutaneous port delivery devices that allow the skin to act as a protective barrier.

■■■ Drug Administration

Since a major principle of i.p. therapy is the delivery of the agent to all regions of the peritoneal cavity, it is important that the drug be administered in sufficient volume to optimize chances that this goal will be attained. In general, most investigators have employed a 2-L treatment volume to deliver i.p. therapy, although in some individuals 3 L or even 4 L may be more appropriate. The drug can either be delivered directly in the 2-L volume, or treatment can be administered in the first liter, with a subsequent liter of fluid added to ensure optimal distribution. The type of fluid to be employed will depend on the specific characteristics of the drug to be administered. For cisplatin, normal saline is appropriate.

If it is not possible to administer at least 2 L into the abdominal cavity, or if the patient complains of significant discomfort with even limited volume, it is likely the fluid is in a small or large pocket, interfering with optimal distribution.

■■■ *Efficacy*

A number of drugs have been examined for their potential efficacy when delivered by the i.p. route in the management of ovarian cancer. Because of its central role in the management of this disease, cisplatin has been the agent most carefully examined for i.p. administration.

Several studies have shown that approximately 20% to 30% of previously treated ovarian cancer patients will achieve a surgically documented response to i.p. cisplatin. However, responses are essentially limited to a small subset of patients in this clinical setting.

In the experience of Memorial Sloan-Kettering Cancer Center investigators (Table 5.2), the surgically defined complete response rate is approximately 35% to 40% for patients who have demonstrated a response to front-line cisplatin or carboplatin-based systemic therapy but who persist in having either microscopic disease or very small-volume macroscopic tumor (largest residual mass less than 0.5 cm in maximum diameter) at second-look laparotomy. However, for patients who have failed to exhibit a response to platinum-

■■■ Table 5.2

Surgically Documented Complete Response Rates to Salvage I.P. Cisplatin Based on Maximum Tumor Diameter and Prior Response to Systemic Cisplatin*

	Maximum Tumor Diameter	
	<0.5–1 cm	**>1 cm**
Prior response to systemic cisplatin		
Yes	35%–40%	<10%
No	<10%	0%

* Experience of Memorial Sloan-Kettering Cancer Center.

based systemic therapy (even if they have small-volume residual disease), or where any tumor mass exceeds 0.5 to 1 cm in maximum diameter, the surgically defined complete response rate is less than 10%.

Several points can be made about these observations, which have been confirmed by other investigators. First, as strongly suggested by preclinical studies showing the limited penetration of drugs directly into tumor or normal tissue, the only patients who have a realistic opportunity to benefit from i.p. treatment are those with very small-volume disease present when treatment is initiated. Second, any added benefit from the high local drug concentrations achieved within the peritoneal cavity following regional drug delivery will likely be "relative" rather than "absolute." Thus, for a patient whose tumor has progressed through systemically delivered cisplatin (i.e., tumor inherently "drug resistant"), it is highly unlikely that the 10- to 20-fold increased concentrations found within the peritoneal cavity after i.p. administration can be translated into major clinical benefit. However, for those patients who have exhibited a significant antitumor response (i.e., tumor inherently "drug sensitive") but who persist in having small-volume residual disease, it is possible the high concentrations of the drug in direct contact with the tumor can achieve additional clinically relevant tumor cell kill.

Antitumor activity has been shown after other drugs including carboplatin, paclitaxel, α-interferon, and γ-interferon have been delivered by the i.p. route as second-line therapy to patients with ovarian cancer. However, the relative efficacy of these drugs cannot be assessed on the basis of the available data.

The experience to date with i.p. therapy leads to the conclusion that there are several situations where this therapeutic strategy is a rational approach in the management of ovarian cancer (Table 5.3). Randomized trial data have revealed that the administration of i.p. cisplatin as a component of primary chemotherapy results in superior survival,

■■■■ **Table 5.3**
*Clinical Situations Where I.P. Therapy Is a Rational Therapeutic
Option to Consider in the Management of Ovarian Cancer*

1. *Salvage therapy* of small-volume residual disease (microscopic only or <0.5-cm maximum diameter macroscopic tumor)
2. *Consolidation therapy* of patients with advanced, high-grade cancer who attain a surgical CR (ultimate relapse rate, 50%–60%)
3. *Primary therapy* of high-risk low-stage ovarian cancer (e.g., stage 1C, stage II)
4. *Primary therapy* of advanced ovarian cancer along with, or immediately after systemic drug delivery

compared with intravenous cisplatin, in women with small-volume residual advanced ovarian cancer.

■■■■ *Complications*

■■■■ Chemotherapy Complications

Toxicities associated with i.p. chemotherapy can either be systemic or local. For drugs that are not limited by their local side effects after i.p. administration (including cisplatin, carboplatin, and the interferons), dose-limiting toxicity will be the systemic effects of the agents. For example, the major difficulties associated with i.p. cisplatin administration include emesis, neurotoxicity, and renal insufficiency, whereas for carboplatin the principal side effect is bone marrow suppression.

However, for agents associated with the local toxicity (including paclitaxel, mitoxantrone, doxorubicin, and mitomycin C), systemic side effects are uncommon. The most common local toxicity is abdominal pain (which can be severe) due to peritoneal cavity irritation and inflammation. This can lead to the development of adhesion formation and bowel obstruction. Agents known to be severe irritants or vesicants are not good candidates for i.p. drug delivery. Although pain medications may reduce the severity of discomfort, they will have no impact on the underlying inflammatory process and subsequent adhesion formation.

■ Catheter Complications

Complications can develop during catheter placement (see Access to the Peritoneal Cavity), or may occur after the successful insertion of the delivery device. In a patient with significant adhesions, a catheter may become plastered against the bowel wall and with time erode into the intestinal lumen. Fortunately, this is uncommon, but it is a serious complication of treatment and the catheter must be removed.

A common catheter complication is the formation of a "one-way valve," whereby it is possible to administer the treatment volume without difficulty, but fluid cannot be removed. This is likely due to the formation of a fibrous sheath around the catheter tip. In general, as long as the fluid freely flows into the peritoneal cavity, the development of a one-way valve should not interfere with an i.p. strategy because the treatment volume can usually be allowed to absorb on its own.

Selected Reading

Alberts D, Lin PY, Hannigan EV, et al: Intraperitoneal cisplatin plus intravenous cyclophosphamide versus intravenous cisplatin plus intravenous cyclophosphamide for stage III ovarian cancer. *N Engl J Med* 1996; 335:1950–1955.

Barakat R, Sabbatini P, Bhaskaran D, et al: Intraperitoneal chemotherapy for ovarian carcinoma: Results of long-term follow-up. *J Clin Oncol* 2002; 20:694–698.

Markman M: Intraperitoneal chemotherapy in the management of malignant disease. *Expert Rev Anticancer Ther* 2001; 1:142–148.

Markman M, Reichman B, Hakes T, et al: Responses to second-line cisplatin-based intraperitoneal therapy in ovarian cancer: Influence of a prior response to intravenous cisplatin. *J Clin Oncol* 1991; 9:1801–1805.

Markman M, Bundy BN, Alberts DS, et al: Phase III trial of standard-dose intravenous cisplatin plus paclitaxel versus moderately high-dose carboplatin followed by intravenous paclitaxel and intraperitoneal cisplatin in small-volume stage III ovarian carcinoma: An Intergroup study of the Gynecologic Oncology Group, Southwestern Oncology Group, and Eastern Cooperative Oncology Group. *J Clin Oncol* 2001; 19:1001–1007.

6

VENOUS ACCESS

ANDREW W. MENZIN
AND THOMAS P. MORRISSEY

▰▰▰ Introduction and Indications

The importance of venous access in the management of oncologic patients cannot be overstated. Fluid and blood product delivery, nutritional support, chemotherapy administration, antibiotic therapy, and blood collection are facilitated by the placement of venous catheters. During the course of therapy, however, peripheral veins become either fibrotic or fragile, making cannulation progressively more difficult for the physician or nurse and more traumatic, physically and psychologically, for the patient. The use of central venous catheters provides a long-term solution to these problems.

▰▰▰ Catheter Types

▰▰▰ Peripheral Intravenous Devices

Peripheral intravenous devices may terminate in either peripheral or central veins. They can be placed using aseptic technique in the outpatient setting or in a hospital unit. The duration of use ranges from several days to months, depending on the particular device used.

Peripheral intravenous devices are indicated for short-term access needs. Site selection should be based on several factors, including patient comfort, ease of medication delivery, and prevention of infiltration or extravasation injury.

Chemotherapy of Gynecologic Cancers: Society of Gynecologic Oncologists Handbook 2e, edited by Stephen C. Rubin, MD, Lippincott Williams & Wilkins, Philadelphia © 2004.

Large peripheral veins are optimal. Avoidance of the ante-cubital fossa, if possible, is warranted because large quanti-ties of extravasated fluid can accumulate at this site before clinical signs appear. Venipuncture attempts should begin distally and advance to more proximal sites. A 20-gauge catheter is usually sufficient for the administration of most fluids (including blood products) needed by cancer pa-tients. Catheters should be removed and sites changed after 48 to 72 hours. Chemotherapy is best administered through catheters in place for fewer than 24 hours to ensure integrity of the insertion site. Vesicants should never been infused unless blood return is demonstrated and infusion of saline is tolerated without pain or extravasation.

PERIPHERALLY INSERTED CENTRAL CATHETERS

Peripherally inserted central catheters (PICC) are used for the same indications as other central catheters but are not recommended for rapid or high-volume infusion. PICCs are placed into the veins of the antecubital fossa (cephalic, basilic, or median cubital veins) and extend into the supe-rior vena cava. Simplified insertion technique, avoidance of pneumothorax, and lower infection rates are advantages, but phlebitis, occlusion, and mechanical complications (mi-gration and embolization) are relatively common. Self-care may be difficult.

▬▬ Central Venous Catheters

In 1971, Broviac introduced central venous catheters for the administration of parenteral nutritional support. Following the introduction of the Hickman catheter in 1975, these de-vices have been used in a wide variety of clinical settings. Placement of these lines should be performed in an operat-ing room to ensure appropriate sterile insertion. A variety of catheter types are available (Table 6.1).

TUNNELED CATHETERS

Tunneled catheters are manufactured from silastic and are composed of intravascular, subcutaneous, and external seg-

▬▬ **Table 6.1**
Central Venous Catheters

Tunneled	
Broviac (Davol)	2.7–6.6 French, 71–90 cm in length, single or double lumen with an open end, often used in pediatric patients.
Hickman (Davol)	9.6 French, 65–90 cm, single, double, or multilumen with an open lumen.
Groshong (Davol)	3.5–9.5 French, single or double lumen with a closed end. A valve mechanism allows infusion, aspiration, and closure of the system.
Leonard (Davol)	10.0 French, 90 cm, dual lumen, similar to Hickman.
Implantable	
Hickman (Davol)	Single or double lumen.
Groshong (Davol)	Single or double lumen.
Infus-a-port (Infusaid)	First totally implantable device (1982), single or double lumen.
Port-a-cath (Pharmacia)	Single or double lumen.
Chemo Port (HDC)	Single lumen.
PICC	
Groshong (Davol)	3–5 French, single or dual lumen.
Port-a-catch (Pharmacia)	Single or double lumen.
Infus-a-port (Infusaid)	Single or double lumen.

Modified from Merrick, HW: Venous access, infusion, and perfusion. In: RT Skeel (ed.), Handbook of Cancer Chemotherapy, 3rd ed. Little, Brown and Company, Boston, p. 514.

ments (Figure 6.1), with single or multiple lumens. The presence of an external connecting segment facilitates manipulation for use, but self-care is more intensive, limitations on certain activities exist, and body image is markedly altered. External catheters also carry a higher risk of infection than do totally implanted devices.

IMPLANTABLE DEVICES

Implantable devices employ subcutaneous ports manufactured from titanium or stainless steel attached to single- or

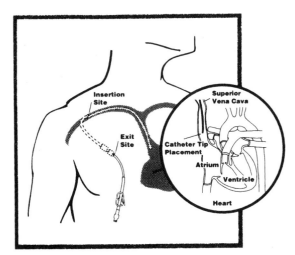

Figure 6.1.
Diagram of tunneled catheter placement.

multiple-lumen catheters. Access is with a noncoring (Huber) needle through a self-sealing silicone single or dual septum (Figure 6.2). Septae will remain intact for approximately 1,000 punctures when a 19-gauge noncoring needle is used, and 2,000 punctures when a 22-gauge noncoring

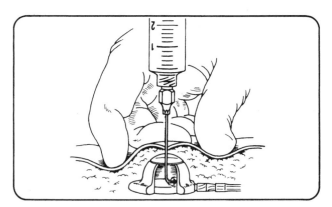

Figure 6.2.
Diagram of a port accession.

needle is selected. Disadvantages of tunneled catheters are avoided, but accessing the port requires more technical skill.

Placement of these implanted ports can be performed in the operating room or by using fluoroscopic or ultrasound guidance in a radiologic procedure suite. In patients with abnormal anatomy, morbid obesity, history of central venous access, or preexisting pulmonary compromise, radiologic guidance can decrease the risk of complications related to placement of central venous catheters.

■■■■ Routine Catheter Care

Exit sites on tunneled catheters should be checked daily for signs of infection. Catheters are to be flushed each day when in use with heparinized saline (100 U/mL). Flushing is required daily to weekly when external catheters are not in regular use. Groshong catheters, because of their closed-valve construction, need to be flushed only with saline on a daily to weekly schedule when used infrequently.

Implanted ports should be flushed monthly with either heparin or saline, depending on the type of catheter attached to the reservoir. Exit site care is eliminated, and dressings are unnecessary.

PICC maintenance is similar to that for the tunneled catheters. Flushing is performed daily.

■■■■ Complications and Their Management

■■■■ Blockage

Blockage of venous catheters may occur secondary to obstruction from blood clots, fibrin sheath formation, lipid deposition, or mineral or medication crystallization. The diagnosis of catheter blockage may be suspected when blood return is not possible, despite the antegrade flow of fluids. This circumstance may result from a flap of material at the catheter opening, or from the catheter tip lying against the blood vessel wall. Having the patient change position and/or follow one of several breathing maneuvers (e.g., deep inspirations, Valsalva) can sometimes distinguish the two occurrences. Blockage is likely if neither antegrade nor retrograde flow is possible. Careful inspection or a chest radiograph can rule out the possibility that the catheter is kinked. In equivocal cases, a catheter dye study may be obtained.

A determination of the likely cause of the blockage will guide the choice of therapy. If a blood clot or fibrin sheath is suspected, the use of a thrombolytic agent is recommended. Streptokinase or urokinase have both been used with success. Streptokinase has been associated with hypersensitivity reaction in up to 15% of patients and requires the formation of a complex with plasminogen or plasmin for activity. Urokinase causes allergic symptoms in only about 2% of cases and does not require complex formation for fibrinolytic activity. Urokinase (5,000 IU [1 mL]) is injected into the occluded catheter or lumen. After 30 minutes to 1 hour, residual solution and obstructing tissue are aspirated. This may be repeated four times within a 24-hour period as needed. Salvage use of tissue plasminogen activator has been successful when other agents have failed. Though systemic effects of these medications are minimized by administration techniques, potential hemorrhagic complications should be considered.

The use of low-dose warfarin (1 mg/day) has been shown in some centers to decrease the risk of catheter malfunction due to thrombosis. This dosage does not prolong prothrombin time in most patients, and in some studies has reduced the observed catheter malfunction rate significantly. However, caution should be used with patients who are nutritionally depleted or receiving certain chemotherapeutic regimens, prolonged use of low-dose warfarin can cause clinically significant prolongation of prothrombin time and bleeding complications.

If occlusion is secondary to lipid deposition, as may be the case in patients on lipid-containing parenteral nutrition, ethyl alcohol may restore patency. Approximately 1 mL of 70% ethyl alcohol is injected and allowed to remain for 1 or

2 hours. Aspiration of the remaining solution and lipid clears the blockage in nearly 80% of catheters.

Occlusion from mineral or medication precipitation can also occur. Management of these types of blockage centers on improving the solubility of the causative agent. This is usually accomplished through pH alteration. Occlusion from medications whose solubility improves in an acid environment may be treated by a dilute solution of hydrochloric acid (0.1 N HCl). Examples include calcium phosphate, heparin, vancomycin, certain β-lactam antibiotics, and aminoglycosides. Approximately 1 mL is injected into the catheter and allowed to remain for 1 hour. Residual solution is then aspirated along with any obstructing material. A febrile episode may accompany the HCl administration, though this occurrence is variable. When basic medications are suspected as the cause, such as other β-lactam antibiotics or phenytoin, the administration of sodium bicarbonate may clear the blockage. About 1 mL of 1-mEq/mL $NaHCO_3$ is injected. Aspiration is performed after 1 hour as described above. If altering the pH in one direction is unsuccessful, empiric treatment with the other solution is a reasonable alternative. Metabolic abnormalities are unusual given the small volumes used and the aspiration of residual solution after administration.

■■■■ Infection

Infection related to both peripheral and central catheters is a concern and a potential cause of significant morbidity and even mortality. Hundreds of thousands of central venous catheters are placed annually, and more than 50,000 access-related infections (ARIs) occur yearly in the United States alone.

MANAGEMENT OF AN ACCESS-RELATED INFECTION

Symptoms of ARIs may be those of local or systemic illness, depending on the site of infection. Infections are classified as tunnel infections, exit site infections, port pocket infections, and device-related bacteremia (DRB). Local signs are typical of the first three types, with aspiration of purulent material likely (though not mandatory for the diagnosis of a tunnel infection). DRB may be defined specifically with regard to results from a catheter tip culture or quantitative blood cultures. The latter criteria require (1) greater than 10 times more colony-forming units (CFU) of bacteria per milliliter in blood drawn from the affected device than found in peripherally obtained blood specimens, or (2) greater than 1,000 CFU in blood drawn through the device, when peripheral specimens are negative.

Given the expected route of inoculation due to migration of bacteria from the skin along the catheter, common organisms isolated are typical cutaneous flora, primarily coagulase-negative staphylococci (e.g., *Staphylococcus epidermidis*) and *Staphylococcus aureus*. The possibility of hematogenous seeding as a cause of ARI is suggested when enteric Gram-negative organisms or fungi are identified. Contaminated solutions may also give rise to an ARI. Specific organisms, such as *Malassezia furfur*, may be associated with certain types of infusions (e.g., lipid-rich parenteral nutrition).

Antibiotic therapy should begin broadly, covering likely cutaneous agents and possible hematogenously derived organisms. After culture results have been obtained, focused treatment reduces the risks of bacterial resistance, antibiotic-related toxicities, and excessive cost. The issue of catheter removal is paramount. DRB may often be treated without catheter removal with good success. However, in the setting of persistent infection, isolation of fungal or certain bacterial organisms (e.g., *Pseudomonas*), or clinical deterioration, catheter removal is recommended. Port pocket and tunnel infections may need to be drained, and this often mandates catheter removal.

PREVENTION OF AN ACCESS-RELATED INFECTION

Table 6.2 summarizes the risk factors that may predict the emergence of ARIs. The cornerstone of prevention of ARIs

▬▬ Table 6.2
Risk Factors for Access-Related Infections

Duration and site of access
Device construction
Techniques of insertion and subsequent management
Underlying acute and chronic medical conditions of the patient

---

is meticulous attention to detail at the time of insertion and during subsequent daily care. Plastic adhesives are less desirable than gauze dressings because of their tendency to accumulate moisture. Although detailed discussions regarding prevention of infection can be found in the selected readings, several points are notable. The use of catheters that are impregnated with minocycline, rifampin, chlorhexidine, or silver sulfadiazine reduces the rate of ARI blood infections. Subcutaneous cuffs do not decrease ARI rates. The use of antibiotic ointments not only fails to decrease infection rates, but is also associated with a greater number of fungal and resistant bacterial infections. The lumen number does not predict the risk of infection, and the choice of a device should be based upon the needs of the patient. Subclavian sites are associated with lower risk of ARI than are jugular lines, presumably because of the increased number of tissue planes that potential infectious agents need to traverse. Ports are less of an infectious risk than are external catheters because the cutaneous barrier is intact and self-care is simpler.

▬▬ Catheter Repair

Specific kits are available from product manufacturers for repair of damaged catheters. Before any catheter is repaired, however, one should consider the alternative of removal and replacement.

Selected Reading

Garrison RN, Wilson MA: Intravenous and central catheter infections. *Surg Clin North Am* 1994; 74:557–570.

Groeger JS, Lucas AB, Coit D: Venous access in the cancer patient. In VT DeVita Jr., S Hellman, SA Rosenberg (eds.), *Cancer: Principles and Practice of Oncology—Updates.* 1991, pp. 1–14.

McGee DC, Gould MK: Preventing complications of central venous catheterization. *N Engl J Med* 2003; 348:1123–1133.

Neiderhuber JE, Ensimenger W Gynes JW, et al: Totally implanted venous and arterial access system to replace external catheters in cancer treatment. *Surgery* 1982; 92:706–712.

Wachs T, Watkins S, Hickman RO: "No more pokes": A review of parenteral access devices. *Nutr Support Serv* 1987; 7:12–18.

PREMEDICATION OF THE CHEMOTHERAPY PATIENT

CHRISTINA S. CHU

Before treatment, evaluation of potential chemotherapy-associated toxicity requires prudent consideration. Adequate premedication may avert or diminish difficult symptoms, as well as irreversible end-organ damage. Many agents commonly used in the treatment of gynecologic malignancies may be associated with severe avoidable toxicities. This chapter will focus on methods to minimize the severity of nausea and emesis, renal and urinary tract toxicity, and hypersensitivity to chemotherapy.

Antiemetic Therapy

Of the various side effects of chemotherapy, nausea and vomiting are among the two most dreaded by patients. The majority of patients undergoing chemotherapy experience nausea and vomiting, and up to 40% may also experience anticipatory symptoms. Though exact mechanisms of chemotherapy-induced nausea and vomiting are poorly defined, most chemotherapies appear to stimulate the chemoreceptor trigger zone in the area postrema of the brain to secrete neurotransmitters such as dopamine, serotonin, and histamine, which in turn activate the neighboring vomiting center to induce nausea and emesis. Other mechanisms may include stimulation of serotonin receptors in the gastrointestinal tract, direct cerebral action, and psychogenic effects.

Chemotherapy of Gynecologic Cancers: Society of Gynecologic Oncologists Handbook 2e, edited by Stephen C. Rubin, MD, Lippincott Williams & Wilkins, Philadelphia © 2004.

Three patterns of emesis have been identified in patients receiving antineoplastic therapy. Acute emesis has been arbitrarily defined as occurring within the first 24 hours after administration of chemotherapy, with delayed emesis occurring more than 24 hours later. Acute emesis is usually most severe, typically peaking 6 or 7 hours after exposure. Delayed emesis may begin as soon as 16 to 24 hours after chemotherapy, and may persist 72 to 96 hours. Anticipatory emesis is a conditioned response that occurs in patients with previously poorly controlled symptoms, and may be experienced by patients before, during, or after chemotherapy administration.

The major categories of antiemetics utilized in premedication regimens are summarized in Table 7.1. Because chemotherapeutic agents engender a range of emetogenicity (Table 7.2), selection of premedications should be tailored to suit the type of chemotherapies to be administered. Dose, route, and schedule of administration may all affect the degree of symptoms experienced by the patient.

██████ Table 7.1
Antiemetics Commonly Used in Premedication Regimens

Class	Drug	Dose
5-HT^3 receptor antagonist	Ondansetron	8–24 mg/PO
	Granisetron	10 mcg/kg; 2 mg PO
	Dolasetron	1.8 mg/kg; 100 mg; 100 mg PO
Substance P/NK$_1$ receptor antagonist	Aprepitant	125 mg PO
Motility agent	Metoclopramide	2–3 mg/kg 20–40 mg PO
Phenothiazine	Prochlorperazine	10 mg i.v./i.m./PO 25 mg PR 15 mg spansule
Benzodiazepine	Lorazepam	0.5–2 mg PO/SL
Corticosteroid	Dexamethasone	8–20 mg

■■ Table 7.2
Emetogenicity of Commonly Used Chemotherapeutics

Frequency of Emesis	Agent
>90%	Cisplatin (>50 mg/m^2)
	Cyclophosphamide (>1,500 mg/m^2)
60–90%	Carboplatin
	Cisplatin (<50 mg/m^2)
	Cyclophosphamide (750–1500 mg/m^2)
	Dactinomycin (>1.5 mg/m^2)
	Doxorubicin (>60 mg/m^2)
	Irinotecan
	Melphalan (i.v.)
	Methotrexate (>1,000 mg/m^2)
30–60%	Cyclophosphamide (<750 mg/m^2)
	Dactinomycin (<1.5 mg/m^2)
	Doxorubicin (20–60 mg/m^2)
	Ifosfamide
	Methotrexate (250–1,000 mg/m^2)
10–30%	Docetaxel
	Doxorubicin (<20 mg/m^2)
	Etoposide
	Fluorouracil (<1,000 mg/m^2)
	Gemcitabine
	Methotrexate (50–250 mg/m^2)
	Paclitaxel
	Topotecan
<10% frequency	Bleomycin
	Hydroxyurea
	Melphalan (PO)
	Methotrexate (<50 mg/m^2)

Adapted from Hesketh PJ, Kris MG, Grunberg SM, et al. Proposal for classifying the acute emetogenecity of cancer chemotherapy. *J Clin Oncol* 1997; 15:103–109.

■■ Highly Emetogenic Chemotherapy

Highly emetogenic chemotherapies include cisplatin and high dose cyclophosphamide. Cisplatin, particularly in doses greater than 50 mg/m^2, may induce both acute and delayed vomiting. Acute emesis may occur within 1 hour of administration, with delayed symptoms lasting 3 to 5 days.

Symptoms appear to be dose related, and prolonged infusion may decrease nausea and vomiting. Cyclophosphamide, at doses greater than 1,500 mg/m^2, is also considered highly emetogenic. Aggressive premedication should be administered approximately 30 minutes before infusion of these agents (Table 7.3). Common antiemetic regimens combine use of a 5-HT^3 receptor antagonist, such as ondansetron (24 mg i.v.), granisetron (10 μg/kg i.v.), or dolasetron (1.8 mg/kg i.v. or 100 mg i.v.), with intravenous dexamethasone (20 mg). Intravenous lorazepam (1–2 mg) or oral aprepitant (125 mg) may also be added.

Continuous infusions of 5-HT^3 antagonists may be used for patients with refractory nausea and vomiting. An example of such a regimen would be a 24-hour infusion of 25 mg ondansetron in 250 mL of D$_5$W. This infusion may be combined with other agents such as corticosteroids, benzodiazepines, or metoclopramide. The use of metoclopramide may occasionally precipitate acute dystonic reactions consisting of torticollis, trismus, or neck retraction. These symptoms may be effectively treated with diphenhydramine 50 mg i.v. or PO.

▆▆▆▆ Moderately Emetogenic Chemotherapy

Several chemotherapies commonly used in the treatment of gynecologic cancers are classified as moderately emetogenic. At lower doses, cisplatin (less than 50 mg/m^2) and cy-

▆▆▆▆ Table 7.3
Premedication Regimens for the Prevention of Acute Phase Emesis

Emesis Risk	Agents
High	5-HT^3 antagonist plus dexamethasone plus lorazepam or 5-HT^3 antagonist plus dexamethasone plus aprepitant
Moderate	5-HT^3 antagonist and/or dexamethasone
Low	Single agents (5-HT^3 antagonist, corticosteroid, dopamine antagonist, phenothiazine, butyrophenone)

clophosphamide (750–1,500 mg/m^2) are considered moderately emetogenic. In addition to acute symptoms, carboplatin may also be associated with significant delayed symptoms, lasting 2 or 3 days after infusion. Symptoms associated with doxorubicin infusion may be attenuated with prolongation of the infusion. Other agents such as methotrexate (>1,000 mg/m^2), ifosfamide, and high-dose fluorouracil are also considered moderately emetogenic. These chemotherapy regimens may be premedicated with a 5-HT^3 antagonist, such as ondansetron (8–24 mg i.v. or PO), granisetron (10 μg/kg i.v. or 2 mg PO), or dolasetron (1.8 mg/kg i.v., 100 mg i.v., or 100 mg PO), in combination with dexamethasone (8–20 mg i.v. or PO).

■■■ Mildly Emetogenic Chemotherapy

Mildly emetogenic drugs include methotrexate, bleomycin, etoposide, gemcitabine, paclitaxel, docetaxel, and liposomal doxorubicin. These agents may be premedicated with single-agent antiemetics. Appropriate choices include dexamethasone (8 mg PO/i.v.), ondansetron (8 mg PO/i.v.), granisetron (10 μg/kg i.v. or 2 mg PO), dolasetron (1.8 mg/kg i.v., 100 mg i.v., or 100 mg PO), metoclopramide (2 mg/kg i.v. or 20 mg PO), prochlorperazine (10 mg i.v./PO), or lorazepam (1–2 mg i.v./PO).

■■■ Regimens for Prophylaxis of Delayed Emesis

Despite adequate treatment for acute emesis associated with chemotherapy administration, a substantial number of patients may experience delayed symptoms 24 to 72 hours later, particularly in association with cisplatin, carboplatin, cyclophosphamide, and doxorubicin. Although nausea and vomiting in the delayed setting may be less severe than acute symptoms, a patient's nutrition and hydration status may still be compromised, and adequate prophylaxis is warranted.

Effective regimens for the prevention of delayed emesis are detailed in Table 7.4. Commonly used regimens include a brief course of dexamethasone in combination with either

████ Table 7.4
Postchemotherapy Regimens for the Prevention of Delayed Emesis

---

- Dexamethasone (8 mg PO BID × 2 days, then 4 mg PO BID × 2 days)
     plus
          metoclopramide (40 mg PO QID × 2 or 3 days)[a]
          or
          5-HT[3] antagonist
               Ondansetron (8 mg PO BID-TID × 2 or 3 days)
               Granisetron (1 mg PO BID OR 2 mg PO QD × 2 or 3 days)
- 5-HT[3] antagonist PO × 2 or 3 days
- Dexamethasone (8 mg PO QD × 3 days) plus aprepitant (80 mg PO QD × 3 days)[b]

---

[a] Because of the risk of dystonic reactions, patients should be advised to take 50 mg diphenhydramine PO at the first sign of symptoms.
[b] If used for delayed vomiting, the 125-mg dose should also be used prechemotherapy in conjunction with corticosteroids and 5-HT[3] antagonists.

metoclopramide or a 5-HT[3] antagonist; single-agent therapy with a 5-HT[3] antagonist; or dexamethasone and a substance P/NK$_1$ antagonist, such as aprepitant.

████ *Prophylaxis for Hypersensitivity Reactions*

Most chemotherapeutics may be associated with hypersensitivity reactions, though few cause reactions in greater than 5% of treated patients. Among the agents used in the treatment of gynecologic malignancies, taxanes and platinum compounds induce the most commonly encountered reactions. Other agents with occasional reports of hypersensitivity include bleomycin, doxorubicin, etoposide, cyclophosphamide, ifosfamide, methotrexate, melphalan, and fluorouracil.

████ Taxanes

Paclitaxel is an antimicrotubule agent that was initially extracted from the bark of the Pacific yew tree. Currently produced semisynthetically, paclitaxel and the related compound docetaxel may be associated with severe hypersensitivity reactions that may in some cases, prove to be dose limiting. In phase 1 trials, the incidence of severe hypersensitivity reactions to paclitaxel was approximately 30%. However, with adequate prophylaxis, the incidence is less than 10%. Because of its poor solubility in water, paclitaxel is formulated in Cremophor EL, a polyoxyethylated castor oil. Initially, allergy to Cremophor EL was thought to be the main cause of hypersensitivity; however, docetaxel has been noted to cause a similar incidence of reactions, despite its formulation in Tween 80 instead of Cremophor EL. With the recommended corticosteroid premedication, the incidence of hypersensitivity to docetaxel has been reported to be about 2% or 3% for those receiving doses of 75 to 100 mg/m^2. Hypersensitivity at the 60-mg/m^2 dose is rare, even in the absence of prophylaxis.

Patients experiencing hypersensitivity typically present with signs and symptoms consistent with a type I allergic reaction: wheezing, dyspnea, urticaria, erythroderma, and agitation. Patients may also experience chest pain, back pain, tachycardia, hypotension, or hypertension. Fatal cardiac arrest has been reported. Onset of symptoms usually occurs within the first few minutes of infusion. Although some patients have reported reactions with later doses, more than 70% occur with the first dose. Longer intervals of paclitaxel infusion have been associated with a decreased incidence of hypersensitivity.

The occurrence of hypersensitivity does not preclude further treatment with the agent. The infusion should be discontinued at the first sign or symptom of reaction. Intravenous normal saline (NS) and additional diphenhydramine should be administered. The vast majority of patients will be able to complete the infusion without additional symptoms after a 30-minute delay. However, for patients who experience a second reaction after reinitiation of the infusion, systematic desensitization to paclitaxel has been successfully utilized in almost all individuals.

Premedication for both paclitaxel and docetaxel are indicated (Table 7.5). Although premedication may not prevent hypersensitivity in all cases, symptoms are generally less severe. As prophylaxis before paclitaxel administration, patients generally receive a combination of corticosteroids, H_1 and H_2 receptor antagonists. Prophylaxis may consist of 20 mg of oral dexamethasone both the night before and the morning of treatment, with intravenous dexamethasone (20 mg), plus diphenhydramine (25–50 mg), and cimetidine (300 mg) given 30 minutes before paclitaxel infusion. If the first cycle of treatment is well tolerated without signs of allergy, subsequent cycles may be preceded by equivalent oral instead of intravenous doses. Patients receiving docetaxel may be premedicated with oral dexamethasone (8 mg BID) starting 1 day before infusion, and continuing for 2 days after infusion. H_1 and H_2 antagonists are not required.

Patients receiving docetaxel may also experience significant peripheral edema. In early phase 2 trials for the treatment of ovarian cancer, in the absence of prophylaxis, 44% to 71% of patients experienced some degree of fluid retention, with 8% to 12% reporting severe symptoms leading to treatment withdrawal. Appropriate corticosteroid prophylaxis may decrease the incidence to approximately 6% in

■■■■ Table 7.5

Prophylaxis for Taxane-associated Hypersensitivity Reactions

Agent	Prophylaxis Regimen
Paclitaxel	Dexamethasone (20 mg PO the night before and morning of infusion[a] *plus* diphenhydramine (25–50 mg i.v.[b] 30 minutes before infusion) *plus* H_2 antagonist (i.v.[b] 30 minutes before infusion: 300 mg cimetidine, 50 mg ranitidine, or 20 mg famotidine)
Docetaxel	Dexamethasone (8 mg PO BID × 3 days starting 1 day before infusion)

[a] May be repeated i.v. 30 minutes before infusion.
[b] If the first cycle of treatment well tolerated, subsequent cycles may be premedicated using oral doses.

those receiving the 100-mg/m^2 dose, and 2% or 3% in those receiving the 75-mg/m^2 dose.

Platinums

Hypersensitivity reactions have also been reported in association with platinum analogues. The reported incidence of cisplatin reactions varies from 5% to 20%, and reactions to carboplatin have been reported to occur in approximately 12% of patients. Several important differences exist between hypersensitivity reactions to platinums and taxanes. Unlike reactions to taxanes, which predominantly present during the initial cycle of treatment, hypersensitivity to platinum compounds typically does not manifest until a significant number of courses have already been administered without any evidence of allergy. In one series, a median of eight platinum courses (cisplatin plus carboplatin) was administered before the observation of an allergic reaction, making hypersensitivity a potential concern during second- or third-line treatment. Patients experiencing a reaction to platinum may also exhibit signs and symptoms that are more subtle than those associated with a taxane reaction, and thus may pass unrecognized. Patients may only report a mild rash or itching several days after chemotherapy. In addition, only half of patients experiencing a carboplatin reaction manifest symptoms within the first few minutes of infusion. Those experiencing severe symptoms may require several hours to achieve resolution.

It should be noted that while prophylaxis for platinum hypersensitivity is not typically recommended, most antiemetic regimens include use of corticosteroids, which may provide some protection from reactions. Patients with mild symptoms, such as rash or itching, may continue treatment with the addition of i.v. diphenhydramine, though infusion may need to be discontinued if symptoms worsen. For severe reactions, such as wheezing or dyspnea, the clinician must decide whether to attempt retreatment with the drug. The relative effectiveness of platinum agents in the treatment of many gynecologic malignancies must be considered against the potential for serious toxicity in this setting. Desensitization to platinum compounds has been reported, with variable success, depending on the severity of symptoms.

▬ Other Agents

Hypersensitivity to other chemotherapeutic agents is rare, and not treated with routine prophylaxis. Allergic reactions to etoposide have been reported in as many as 5% of patients, usually in association with the first exposure to intravenous administration of the drug. Intravenous doxorubicin has also been reported to cause severe type I hypersensitivity. Most other agents commonly in use for the treatment of gynecologic malignancies only cause allergic reactions on a sporadic basis. Methotrexate may induce both type I hypersensitivity as well as type III interstitial pneumonitis. Melphalan and cyclophosphamide, administered both orally and intravenously, may cause type I reactions. Continuous-infusion fluorouracil has been associated with plantar-palmar dermatitis in as many as 30% of patients, and bleomycin has been associated with fever due to release of endogenous pyrogens, occasionally leading to hypotension and disseminated intravascular coagulation in severe cases. Bleomycin may also induce interstitial pneumonitis. Most type I reactions may be effectively treated with intravenous or oral diphenhydramine, with the addition of intravenous corticosteroids if necessary. In severe cases, epinephrine may be required.

▬ *Prophylaxis of Renal and Urinary Tract Toxicity*

Many chemotherapies and their metabolites undergo renal clearance, rendering the kidneys and urinary tract susceptible to injury. Several agents common in the treatment of gynecologic tumors require special consideration to minimize urinary and nephrotoxicity.

███ Cisplatin

Nephrotoxicity may be a dose-limiting toxicity of cisplatin in as many as 35% of patients, and generally occurs in a dose-related, cumulative fashion. Although the mechanism is not clearly defined, damage primarily occurs in the proximal and distal tubules, leading to an increase in the serum creatinine and decrease in the creatinine clearance, as well as electrolyte wasting of sodium, potassium, magnesium, phosphate, and calcium. Hypomagnesemia is a common sequela of cisplatin administration that may persist for months after treatment, though only 10% of patients display symptoms of dizziness, tetany, muscle weakness, or paresthesia. Although repletion with magnesium sulfate during cisplatin administration is routinely used, hypomagnesemia may not be fully alleviated. Cisplatin-associated hyponatremia occurs in fewer than 10% of patients, and has been reported to cause persistent orthostatic hypotension.

Hydration is crucial to minimizing nephrotoxicity. Adequate prehydration may decrease the incidence of nephrotoxicity to approximately 5%. Hydration provides renal protection through several mechanisms. With adequate fluid volume, cisplatin is diluted in the urine and also spends less time in contact with the urothelium, thereby minimizing tubular injury. In addition, high chloride concentrations afforded in normal saline prehydration may inhibit hydrolysis of cisplatin within the renal tubules, also enhancing renal protection.

Hydration regimens may vary depending on the dose of cisplatin. Common regimens are outlined in Table 7.6. The goal of hydration is to maintain urine output of at least 100 mL/hour for 1 or 2 hours before and 4 to 6 hours after cisplatin infusion. Patients receiving cisplatin at doses greater than 50 mg/m^2 should be hydrated with at least 1 L of 1/2 NS, $D_5$1/2 NS, or NS with 20 mEq potassium chloride and 2 g magnesium sulfate given over the two hours both before and after cisplatin administration. At the treating physician's discretion, and depending on the setting of administration (outpatient or inpatient), hydration may be in-

■■■■ Table 7.6
Common Hydration Regimens for Cisplatin Administration

Cisplatin Dose	Regimen[a]
≤50 mg/m^2	Prehyration: 1 L ½ NS[b] + 10 mEq KCl + 1 g MgSO$_4$ over 1 hr[c]
	Antiemetics
	Cisplatin: administered at ≤1 mg/min + 12.5 g mannitol
	Posthydration: 1 L ½NS[b] + 10 mEq KCl + 1 g MgSO$_4$ over 1 hr
>50 mg/m^2	Prehydration: 1 L ½NS[b] + 20 mEq KCl + 2 g MgSO$_4$ over 2 hr[c]
	Antiemetics
	Cisplatin: administered at ≤1 mg/min + 12.5 g mannitol
	Posthydration: 1 L ½NS[b] + 20 mEq KCl + 2 g MgSO$_4$ over 2 hours

Special Considerations
1. Maintain at least 100-mL/hr urine output for minimum of 1 hr before and 4 hr after chemotherapy
2. Avoid aminoglycosides
3. Output (urine, diarrhea, emesis) >200 mL/hr may require additional hydration

[a] Specified volumes of hydration should be considered the minimum recommended. Additional fluid may be administered at the discretion of the treating physician.
[b] Other acceptable intravenous fluids include NS or D$_5$½NS.
[c] Ten milligrams i.v. furosemide is optional and may be considered when administering 2 or more L of hydration.

creased to 2 L prechemotherapy and postchemotherapy, with the interval of infusion increased to 4 to 6 hours. Cisplatin should be infused at no greater than 1 mg/minute, and should be mixed with 12.5 g mannitol to encourage diuresis. Further diuresis with furosemide 10 mg i.v. is optional. Patients receiving less than 50 mg/m^2 of cisplatin should receive a minimum of 1 L of ½ NS, D$_5$ ½ NS, or NS with 10 mEq potassium chloride and 1 g magnesium sulfate over 1 hour both before and after cisplatin infusion. Additional hydration may be necessary to replace losses due to excessive emesis or diarrhea.

▬▬ Cyclophosphamide and Ifosfamide

Cyclophosphamide and ifosfamide are alkylating agents with similar chemical structures. Both are metabolized to acrolein, which is excreted by the kidneys and may lead to severe hemorrhagic cystitis. However, despite their similarities, only ifosfamide is associated with significant renal toxicity because of its unique effect on renal tubules.

Cyclophosphamide may be administered orally or intravenously, in a variety of different doses and schedules. Patients receiving high-dose i.v. cyclophosphamide ($>3,000$ mg/m^2) in conjunction with stem cell transplant are at highest risk of hemorrhagic cystitis, and require aggressive prehydration and posthydration with frequent bladder emptying. Approximately 40% of these patients may experience microscopic or gross hematuria. Bladder protectants such as mesna should be used in this setting. In those patients at risk for tumor lysis syndrome, i.v. hydration may include bicarbonate to alkalinize the urine. Cystitis is unusual at the lower i.v. doses (less than or equal to 1,000 mg/m^2) more commonly used in the treatment of gynecologic malignancies, and is reported in fewer than 10% of patients. Standard hydration for these doses should be designed to assure urine output of greater than 100 mL/hour, and may consist of 1/2NS or D$_5$1/2NS with potassium chloride infused at a rate of 150 to 200 mL/hour for 2 to 4 hours before infusion. For treatment of epithelial ovarian carcinomas, cyclophosphamide is usually given in conjunction with cisplatin, in which case, hydration before and after cisplatin administration is adequate.

The need for adequate hydration and diuresis must be balanced with the risk for fluid retention. Cyclophosphamide has been associated with an antidiuretic effect, especially at higher doses. Water retention may lead to electrolyte abnormalities, low sodium, and potentially, to seizures and death. Fluid retention may require forced diuresis with furosemide.

Ifosfamide's principle toxicity is also hemorrhagic cystitis, and coadministration with mesna is standard. Mesna dosing regimens vary, but are generally based on the dose of ifosfamide. Patients receiving short infusions of ifosfamide (1 hour) may be treated with a dose 40% to 60% of the ifosfamide dose administered intravenously as a prechemotherapy bolus. Similar doses of mesna should be repeated 4 and 8 hours after completion, administered either intravenously or orally. An acceptable alternative is to use a dose of mesna equal to 100% to 120% the ifosfamide dose infused continuously over 12 hours, beginning 15 minutes before ifosfamide. Patients receiving longer infusions of ifosfamide (12–24 hours) may also be treated with a continuous infusion of mesna dosed at 100% to 120% of the ifosfamide dose. These mesna infusions should be concurrent with ifosfamide administration and continue for 12 hours after completion.

Although mesna administration is effective in limiting bladder toxicity, it is not protective against renal damage. With tubular damage, patients may develop an elevated creatinine and Fanconi syndrome with aminoaciduria, glycosuria, and hypophosphatemia. Although acute renal dysfunction may be reversible, patients may progress to renal failure.

▬ Methotrexate

Methotrexate is an antimetabolite that blocks DNA synthesis through its effects on folate metabolism. The majority of the drug is excreted unchanged in the urine, and may induce renal toxicity via two mechanisms. The drug may produce direct damage of renal tubules, but acidic urine may also lead to precipitation of methotrexate and its metabolites within tubules. Patients receiving high-dose regimens (greater than or equal to 1.5 g/m^2) require adequate intravenous hydration and vigorous diuresis. Alkalinization of the urine with the addition of sodium bicarbonate to the i.v. fluid has also helped to decrease the risk of renal failure.

Suggested Reading

DeVita VT Jr., Hellman S, Rosenberg SA (eds.): *Cancer Principles and Practice of Oncology*, 6th edition. Lippincott Williams &Wilkins, Philadelphia, 2001.

Kaye SB, Piccart M, Aapro M, Francis P, Kavanagh J: Phase II trials of docetaxel (Taxotere) in advanced ovarian cancer—an updated overview. *Eur J Cancer* 1997; 33:2167–2170.

Markman M, Kennedy A, Webster K, Culp B, Peterson G, Belinson J: Paclitaxel-associated hypersensitivity reactions: Experience of the Gynecology Oncology Program of the Cleveland Clinic Cancer Center. *J Clin Oncol* 2000; 18:102–105.

Markman M, Kennedy A, Webster K, Elson P, Peterson G, Kulp B, Belinson J: Clinical Features of hypersensitivity reactions to carboplatin. *J Clin Oncol* 1999; 17:1141.

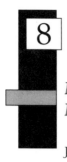

8

MANAGEMENT OF THE NEUTROPENIC PATIENT

JOHN P. CURTIN

Patients receiving cytotoxic chemotherapy for malignancy are at risk for complications related to neutropenia. The definition of neutropenia varies, but generally, grade 3 toxicity is defined as a neutrophil count of less than 1,000 cells/mm^3 and grade 4 toxicity is equivalent to a neutrophil count of less than 500 cells/mm^3. Bone marrow toxicity is one of the more common side effects of cytotoxic chemotherapy and is often the determinant of maximal tolerated dose in phase 1 trials of new chemotherapeutic agents. In phase 2 and 3 clinical trials, one of the leading indications for dose reduction of chemotherapy is neutrophil toxicity.

Neutropenia is common in reports of either single-agent or combination chemotherapy regimens. It is important to remember that although some degree of neutropenia may occur as a consequence of nearly every cytotoxic chemotherapeutic agent, fever associated with neutropenia requiring medical attention is uncommon and documented sepsis is even less common. The recognition of the importance of prompt empiric antibiotic coverage for the patient who is neutropenic has resulted in a significant decline in the morbidity and mortality of chemotherapy and has allowed for the dose intensification of some agents and the formulation of new, more effective combinations of chemotherapeutic drugs. More recently, the introduction of growth factors has further improved patient care. Although these agents are expensive, their proper use short-

Chemotherapy of Gynecologic Cancers: Society of Gynecologic Oncologists Handbook 2e, edited by Stephen C. Rubin, MD, Lippincott Williams & Wilkins, Philadelphia © 2004.

ens the duration of neutropenia and reduces hospitalization time significantly.

▬ *Pathophysiology and Common Infections*

In the uncompromised patient, there is constant surveillance by the body's natural defense against pathogens. The site of this surveillance is primarily the skin and along mucous membranes. Because the skin and mucous membranes cannot constantly maintain a complete barrier, neutrophils play a crucial role in the prevention of infections. Therefore, when a patient becomes neutropenic, the most common disease-causing pathogens are bacteria normally found either on the skin (i.e., *Staphylococcus epidermis* or *Staphylococcus aureus*) or bacteria from the gastrointestinal tract (i.e., *Escherichia coli* or *Klebsiella pneumoniae*). Patients with significant tumor burden may be at increased risk because of contributing factors, including anemia and malnutrition, both of which impair the normal host response to infection. Other important factors that may contribute to increased morbidity include tumor involvement of the intestinal tract. This may result in partial or complete obstruction with overgrowth of intestinal flora or breakdown of the mucosal barriers, which normally prevent hematogenous seeding of intestinal bacteria. The urinary tract can also be compromised by the local effects of tumor invasion with mucosal erosion and/or obstruction and stasis. Other comorbid factors may include malnutrition, recent surgery, and/or radiation therapy with potential for additive disruption of the natural barriers to bacterial invasion.

Bacteria generally pose the greatest threat to the neutropenic patient during the initial presentation, when the patient becomes symptomatic, especially when the neutrophil count is less than $100/mm^3$. Although the patient may be severely neutropenic, almost all patients will continue to mount a febrile response to any infection. This is often the only clinical sign of a potential problem and must not be ignored. The risk to the patient is that, in the absence of the normal humoral response to bacterial infection mediated by the neutrophils, a simple local infection can evolve within a short period into a life-threatening situation, with sepsis and shock.

Other pathogens may contribute to the initial presentation in the neutropenic patient but do not generally pose a great threat to the patient's life. Commonly, fungal and viral pathogens present a secondary problem in the severely immunocompromised patient. Fungal infections may occur as a secondary infection resulting from overgrowth due to the long-term effects of broad-spectrum antibiotics on the bacteria of the alimentary tract. Viral infections rarely present a significant problem for the patient with neutropenia alone and are commonly associated with pancytopenia for prolonged periods, which is rare in the solid tumors, including gynecologic malignancies.

▬▬ Incidence

The incidence of neutropenia will vary with the agent or agents used, as well as the schedule of administration. Single agents are less likely to cause neutropenia than combination regimens. Two of the more commonly proscribed agents, carboplatin and paclitaxel, are associated with a significantly higher level of myelosuppression than other drugs such as cisplatin and cyclophosphamide. The interval between administration of a myelosuppressive agent and the resulting neutropenia varies from agent to agent an important consideration when planning the schedule of therapy. Carboplatin bone marrow toxicity is usually seen at approximately 17 to 21 days after administration. Paclitaxel bone marrow toxicity is dose and schedule dependent; the most commonly proscribed schedule is a 3-hour infusion. Nadir counts usually occur at 8 to 11 days and recovery of neutropenia precedes the effect of carboplatin.

Paclitaxel does not have a cumulative toxic effect on the bone marrow, and the degree of neutropenia should not be more severe after the initial treatment with paclitaxel.

Patients with solid tumors may be at less risk of neutropenic complications than those patients with hematologic malignancy, such as leukemia, or patients who are status post–bone marrow transplant, because the duration of neutropenia is usually shorter for the patient with a solid tumor. Only a small percentage of patients with grade 3 or 4 neutrophil toxicity (seen in approximately 80% of patients treated with standard doses of carboplatin and paclitaxel) will need medical evaluation or hospitalization for management of fever when neutropenic.

Advanced ovarian cancer is often characterized by recurrent disease treated in sequence with an increasing number of active second line chemotherapeutic agents. Cumulative bone marrow toxicity will frequently be the limiting factor in the use of agents such as topotecan, liposomal doxorubicin, and etoposide.

▬ Initial Evaluation and Management

Many patients will be neutropenic and without symptoms after chemotherapy. Routine serial determinations of complete blood count (CBC) may be a part of a protocol evaluation of a new agent or combinations of different agents. When the patient is found to be neutropenic and is without symptoms, no further workup is indicated. The patient should be given reinforcement advice regarding the importance of notifying the treating physician of any new signs or symptoms. The physician may want to increase the frequency of CBC determinations during the period of neutropenia. Avoidance of crowds and/or contact with individuals with simple infections may be reasonable; however, the greatest risk to the patient remains her own normal bacterial flora. Addition of prophylactic oral antibiotics is not indicated. If the period of neutropenia is known to be short (i.e., less than 4 or 5 days), then addition of granulocyte colony-stimulating factor (G-CSF) is not indicated.

A single oral temperature higher than 38.3°C (101.0°F) or fever of 38°C (100.4°F) that persists for 2 hours is an indication for medical evaluation in any patient receiving chemotherapy. Patients should be advised of this potential complication at the time they start chemotherapy, and a plan should be established for how to seek prompt and timely medical attention. This consideration is especially important if the patient is not geographically close to the medical center where the chemotherapy is administered.

Patients who report fever at home may be afebrile when they present for the initial evaluation; this should not be taken as an indication that a complete workup is unnecessary. A complete examination is critical to proper triage of the patient who is at risk for neutropenia and reports a fever. Vital signs are the first important information obtained. In addition to documenting an elevated temperature, baseline heart rate and blood pressure are noted. An elevated heart rate may be only a manifestation of the febrile state; however, this can also be a sign of the hyperdynamic state of sepsis. Hypotension can also be found on initial evaluation, and the etiology may be related to multiple causes. The prime concern of the initial medical evaluation is to initiate appropriate therapy in a timely manner.

For the patient with any signs of cardiovascular compromise related to an infectious process, broad-spectrum antibiotics should be started immediately after intravenous access is achieved. Equally important is fluid resuscitation and placement of monitoring access, including, at a minimum, a central venous pressure monitor and a Foley catheter to follow urine output. The patient who is suspected to have a shock syndrome should be admitted to an intensive care setting for close monitoring. Persistent hypotension should be treated with pressor agents to maintain perfusion and renal blood flow. If the patient is at risk for staphylococcal sepsis and is exhibiting signs of vascular instability, addition of vancomycin for coverage of staphylococcal species is indicated.

Upon presentation for evaluation, if the patient at risk for neutropenia is found to be hemodynamically stable, an intravenous access is established and blood should be obtained for CBC, blood urea nitrogen/creatine ratio, liver function studies, and serum electrolytes. Urine is obtained for urinalysis and culture. Blood cultures are obtained from peripheral sites and, if the patient has a venous access device, a separate blood culture is obtained from the device and properly labeled. If the patient is found to be febrile and a neutropenic state is strongly suspected (a recent CBC reported neutropenia), antibiotics can be initiated without waiting for laboratory determinations to be available. Before administering any therapy, the patient should be questioned regarding any potential drug allergies.

Once therapy has been initiated, the evaluation of the patient continues with a complete history and physical examination. Recent exposure to any other individuals who were ill is documented. The date of the last course of chemotherapy is recorded with documentation of dose of the agents and the schedule of administration. Symptoms of site-specific complaints are carefully noted. Physical examination is complete with particular attention to potential areas of concern noted during the history. The oropharynx is examined and, if there are signs of inflammation or exudate, a culture is obtained, including fungal and viral. The lungs are examined, as well as the heart. Any new finding of decreased breath sounds, dullness on percussion, or a newly noted heart murmur requires further workup. The abdominal examination focuses on signs of an intraabdominal process, particularly in the patient who is status post–recent laparotomy and chemotherapy. An internal pelvic examination and digital rectal examination are classically taught to be avoided for the neutropenic patient, although there are few data to support this practice. If the neutropenic patient has recently had a hysterectomy, the vaginal examination should be done to evaluate the vaginal cuff and to rule out the possibility of a pelvic cellulitis or a cuff abscess. The perianal area should be visually inspected to determine if there is a possibility of rectal or anal pathology. The extremities are examined with particular attention given to recent infection sites and intravenous access punctures. Recent surgical wounds are a potential site of infection, especially if there is seroma formation or wound separation.

Any positive findings during the initial physical examination warrant further evaluation and culture. Suspicious fluid collections or clinically suspect abscesses should be aspirated and the aspirate sent for culture and sensitivity. An obvious abscess should be drained as soon as the initial antibiotics have been given, allowing for establishment of adequate serum levels of antibiotics. Once the patient has been evaluated, therapy has been initiated, and the patient is determined to be stable, further radiographic tests can be obtained. At a minimum, a two-view chest radiograph is indicated for the febrile neutropenic patient. If the patient has gastrointestinal-related complaints, an abdominal series is also obtained. Abdominal-pelvic computed tomography scans are indicated if there is a possibility of an intraabdominal abscess.

■■■■ Selection of Antibiotics

Selection of antibiotics should follow an established protocol so that all personnel involved in the care of the patient understand the standing orders. Broad-spectrum antibiotics are indicated with special emphasis on agents that provide Gram-negative coverage, since these infections pose the greatest threat to the neutropenic patient (Table 8.1). The efficacy of these empiric regimens was demonstrated in the 1970s, when the principal pathogens were Gram-negative organisms from the gastrointestinal tract. The most life threatening of these infections were due to *Pseudomonas* species, and the antimicrobial agents were selected to provide a high degree of coverage for Gram-negative organisms in general and pseudomonads in particular (Table 8.2). These regimens have evolved from three drug regimens to two drug regimens (combination of an aminoglycoside and either a third-generation cephalosporin or a penicillin derivative with β-lactamase inhibitor) that have been considered to be the standard of care. More recent studies have

■■■■ Table 8.1

Standard Antibiotic Regimens for Empiric Treatment of
Neutropenia and Fever

Single agent
  Cefepime
  Ceftazidime
  Meropenem
Combination
  Ceftazidime *plus* aminoglycoside
  Ticarcillin/clavulanic acid *plus* aminoglycoside
Modifications
  Early discharge
    Stable patient with no focal findings and negative blood cultures
    Discharged with broad-spectrum oral antibiotics
  Persistant fever associated with neutropenia after 3–5 days of empiric
antibiotics
    Add vancomycin if venous catheter infection with *Staphylococcus*
epidermidis is suspected
    Add either fluconazol or liposomal amphotericin B to cover possible
fungal infection

---

focused on monotherapy, reflecting the concern regarding
the use of an aminoglycoside in patients who are receiving
nephrotoxic chemotherapeutic drugs, such as the platin-
based compounds. A recent metaanalysis suggested that
use of single-agent β lactam (third- or fourth-generation

■■■■ Table 8.2

Common Infections in Gynecologic
Oncology Patients (N = 98) Treated for
Febrile Neutropenia

Pathogen	n
Gram-negative organisms	10
Gram-positive organisms	9
Staphylococcus epidermidis	5
Enterococci	2
Candida	1

Positive cultures, N = 27 (27.6%).

cephalosporins or carbapenems) should be regarded as the standard of care.

The increasing utilization of semipermanent venous access catheters has resulted in an increase in the incidence of Gram-positive infections in the neutropenic patient. These infections are not commonly associated with significant sepsis and shock. For this reason, empiric addition of an antibiotic with broad Gram-positive coverage is not indicated in the neutropenic patient with a venous access device, unless the patient presents in an unstable manner, with obvious signs of sepsis.

Although less common in patients with gynecologic cancers, prolonged neutropenia and fever may indicate active fungal or viral infection. Fungal infections are most commonly related to *Candida* or *Aspergillus* species. Typically, these infections occur in profoundly neutropenic patients who have been treated with antibiotics. Mucosal infections do not usually require systemic therapy and will respond to topical treatments. For oral thrush, nystatin solution or clotrimazole troches should be started immediately when antibiotic therapy is initiated. The danger of an untreated mucosal fungal infection is that with prolonged antibiotic treatment, combined with neutropenia and alteration of the normal mucosal barrier, the patient may develop an overwhelming fungal septicemia with significant associated morbidity. In this critical situation, the patient must be treated aggressively with systemic antifungal agents. If the patient remains febrile following 3 or 4 days of empiric antibiotic therapy, empiric antifungal therapy should be started. Standard therapy has been amphotericin B. Liposomal amphotericin B and intravenous fluconazole are two new agents that are equally effective against fungal septicemia; either agent is preferred for fungal infections when the patient is being treated with platin-based agents because of the extreme nephrotoxicity of amphotericin B. Fluconazole may not have the same activity against *Aspergillus* as amphotericin B; individual institution profiles must be considered before deciding on one agent. Fluconazole does have the advantage of an oral formulation allowing for conversion to outpatient therapy.

Viral infections usually represent recrudescence of latent viruses that are common in the general population. Both the herpes simplex and zoster viruses have a dormant state with a tendency to erupt during periods of stress and immunosuppression. Antiviral agents specific for these common pathogens are now available that act to diminish the duration and severity of the acute eruptions. Depending on the status of the patient and ability to take medications orally, the treatment of choice for herpes simplex is 200 mg acyclovir PO or i.v., five times daily. For treatment of herpes zoster, famciclovir has recently been approved as a specific antiherpes agent; acyclovir is also effective. Patients who experience repeated episodes of herpetic lesions benefit from low-dose prophylaxis with oral acyclovir.

■■■■ Duration of Therapy

The standard management of the neutropenic patient has been to continue treatment with systemic antibiotics until the granulocyte count returns to a level above 500 to 1,000 neutrophils/mm^3 and the patient is afebrile. During treatment, the daily routine blood tests should include a CBC, and serum creatinine for the patient receiving an aminoglycoside. Other routine laboratory tests should be ordered on an individual basis depending on the initial values found on admission and the patient's daily progress. Blood cultures and urine cultures are ordered only if the patient continues to remain symptomatic with fever and the initial cultures were negative after 72 hours, or in the event of an acute clinical deterioration. Reculture of the patient who has an initial positive culture is not clinically indicated unless the patient continues to have febrile episodes after 48 to 72 hours of antimicrobial therapy.

Recent studies have focused on outpatient management neutropenic patients at low risk for serious complications. If the patient is stable after 24 hours, has no focal finding (i.e., pneumonia) and preliminary cultures are negative, the patient can be switched to a combination of broad-spectrum oral antibiotics; one study utilized oral ciproflaxin plus amoxicillin-clavulanate. Complete instructions to the patient regarding parameters to be monitored at home and indications for return to the hospital are critical to the successful management of low-risk patients as outpatients.

If the patient remains hospitalized and on therapy, patients should be examined daily, with special emphasis on known or suspected sites of infection. Serial radiographs are indicated for abnormal findings on admission studies. Patients should be monitored for side effects of therapy, including development of allergic reactions to the antimicrobial agents. The manifestation of these hypersensitivity reactions varies by the agents prescribed. Rare side effects include bleeding diathesis due to multifactorial causes. The etiology of bleeding includes thrombocytopenia related to the previous chemotherapy, thrombocytopenia related to the antibiotics, and vitamin K-related bleeding problems due to the depletion of bacteria in the proximal intestine. These complications are rare but, in the already compromised patient, can result in significant morbidity.

Growth Factors

The introduction of bone marrow progenitor cell growth factors has impacted significantly on the management of the neutropenic patient. The two most commonly used agents are G-CSF and granulocyte-macrophage colony-stimulating factor. Both agents are administered subcutaneously and have a rapid effect on the bone marrow. These agents are currently indicated as an adjunct in the management of neutropenia and fever. G-CSF effectively stimulates bone marrow recovery however not all patients are candidates for these agents. These agents are rarely indicated as prophylaxis in the anticipation of neutropenia unless the patient has experienced significant morbidity (i.e., pneumonia, sepsis, and/or fungal infection) during previous cycles. Addition of G-CSF with future regimens may minimize the necessity of subsequent dose reductions in clinically active chemotherapy.

Unless the patient is on a research protocol that prescribes growth factors, routine addition of these agents is not indicated during the first episode of uncomplicated neutropenia and fever. A recent randomized trial found that the use of G-CSF in the management of patients with chemotherapy-induced febrile neutropenia resulted in a decrease in the days of absolute neutropenia and the time to resolution of fever in the G-CSF group; however, length of hospitalization was equal between the G-CSF–treated group and the placebo control group. Subsets that appear to benefit are patients with significant neutropenia (less than 100 cells/mm^3), patients with a documented infection, and patients with an anticipated duration of neutropenia of 7 or more days.

Suggested Reading

Curtin JP, Hoskins WJ, Rubin SC, et al.: Chemotherapy-induced neutropenia and fever in patients receiving cisplatin; based chemotherapy for ovarian malignancy. *Gynecol Oncol* 1991; 40:17–20.

De Pauw BE, Deresinski SC, Feld R, et al.: Ceftazidime compared with piperacillin and tobramycin for the empiric treatment of fever in neutropenic patients with cancer: A multicenter randomized trial. *Ann Intern Med* 1994; 120:834–844.

Havel K, Engert A. Clinical applications of granulocyte colony-stimulating factor: An update and summary. *Ann Hematol* 2003 82:207–213.

Innes HE, Smith DB, O'Reilly SM, et al.: Oral antibiotics with early hospital discharge compared with in-patient intravenous antibiotics for low-risk febrile neutropenia in patients with cancer: a prospective randomized controlled single centre study. *Br J Cancer* 2003; 89:43–49.

Maher DW, Lieschke GJ, Green M, et al.: Filgrastim in patients with chemotherapy-induced febrile neutropenia. *Ann Intern Med* 1994; 121:492–501.

McMeekin DS, Gazzaniga C, Berman M, et al.: Retrospective review of gynecologic oncology patients with therapy induced neutropenic fever. *Gynecol Oncol* 1996; 62:247–253

Paul M, Soares-Weiser K, Leibovici L: β Lactam monotherapy versus β lactam-aminoglycoside combination therapy for fever with neutropenia: Systematic review and meta-analysis. *BMJ* 2003; 326:1111–1120.

Pizzo PA, Hathorn JW, Hiemenz J, et al.: A randomized trial comparing ceftazidime alone with combination antibiotic therapy in cancer patients with fever and neutropenia. *N Engl J Med* 1986; 315:552–558.

Rubin M, Hathorn JW, Marshall D, et al.: Gram-positive infections and the use of vancomycin in 550 episodes of fever and neutropenia. *Ann Intern Med* 1988; 108:30–35.

Wade J: Febrile neutropenia. In MD Abeloff, JO Armitage, AS Lichter, et al. (eds.), *Clinical Oncology,* 2nd edition. Churchill Livingstone, New York, 2000.

Winston DJ, Hanthorn JW, Schuster MG, et al.: A multicenter randomized trial of fluconazol versus amphotericin B for empiric antifungal therapy of febrile neutropenic patients with cancer. *Am J Med* 2000; 108: 282–289.

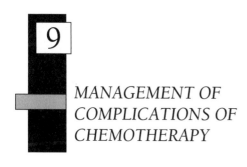

9

MANAGEMENT OF COMPLICATIONS OF CHEMOTHERAPY

YUKIO SONODA AND
RICHARD R. BARAKAT

▓▓▓ *Allergic Reactions*

▓▓▓ Pathophysiology

Nearly all available antitumor agents (Table 9.1) used to treat gynecologic cancer can be associated with hypersensitivity reactions in approximately 5% of patients, although reactions severe enough to be dose-limiting have only been reported for paclitaxel. In phase 1 trials of paclitaxel, anaphylactic-like hypersensitivity reactions were reported to occur in 3% to 28% of treated patients. These initial studies, which used bolus injections or short intravenous infusions, were associated with a high incidence of such reactions, characterized by bronchospasm, dyspnea, stridor, cutaneous flushing, urticaria, and hypotension.

The mechanism responsible for these classic type I hypersensitivity reactions is unclear and may be secondary to paclitaxel or its excipient, Cremophor EL, a nonionic surfactant derived from castor oil used to solubilize paclitaxel. Cremophor EL induces histamine release and has caused similar reactions when used as a vehicle for other drugs, although the amount of Cremophor EL required to solubilize paclitaxel is greater. These reactions occur most commonly with the first or second cycle of drug exposure and occur

Chemotherapy of Gynecologic Cancers: Society of Gynecologic Oncologists Handbook 2e, edited by Stephen C. Rubin, MD, Lippincott Williams & Wilkins, Philadelphia © 2004.

■■■■ Table 9.1
Chemotherapy Agents Used in the
Treatment of Gynecologic Cancers
That Are Associated With
Hypersensitivity Reactions

High Incidence
　Paclitaxel
Low Incidence
　Anthracyclines
　Carboplatin/Cisplatin
　Cyclophosphamide
　Melphalan
　Ifosfamide
　Etoposide
　Fluorouracil
　Methotrexate
　Mitomycin
　Mitoxantrone
　Vinca alkaloids
　Hydroxyurea

within minutes of starting the drug infusion. Paclitaxel-induced hypersensitivity reactions do not seem to be caused solely by IgE directed against paclitaxel or its Cremophor vehicle, as the majority of these episodes occur during the initial treatment. These reactions are, therefore, nonimmunologically mediated by the direct release of histamine and other vasoactive substances from mast cells and basophils, a mechanism similar to reactions caused by iodinated radiocontrast dyes.

■■■■ Management

Initially, hypersensitivity reactions appeared to be indirectly related to the duration of paclitaxel infusion, with some investigators reporting the rates of adverse reactions to be 16%, 13%, and 7% with 3-, 6-, and 24-hour infusions, respectively. Currently, paclitaxel can be safely administered on an outpatient basis via a 3-hour intravenous infusion with prophylactic antiallergic premedications. Premedication has decreased the incidence of acute paclitaxel hypersensitivity reactions to approximately 2%. These regimens are based on those used in patients with allergic reactions to iodinated radiocontrast and include dexamethasone, the H_1 antagonist diphenhydramine, and an H_2 blocker, either cimetidine or ranitidine.

The following pretreatment prophylaxis is recommended before paclitaxel administration:

Dexamethasone: 20 mg PO or i.v., 12 and 6 hours before treatment

Diphenhydramine: 50 mg i.v., 30 minutes before treatment

Cimetidine (or *ranitidine*): 300 mg (or 50 mg) i.v., 30 minutes before treatment

Despite effective premedication, hypersensitivity reactions have not been completely eliminated, and some patients may experience severe reactions. A physician should be present for the first administration of paclitaxel. If an allergic reaction occurs during treatment, the medication must be discontinued immediately and an intravenous line with normal saline should be maintained. Vital signs should be monitored closely and the patient should be observed for signs of respiratory distress. Treatment options include administration of fluids, antihistamines, vasopressors, corticosteroids, and bronchodilators. (Table 9.2)

▌ **Retreatment of Allergic Patients**

There is increasing evidence that some patients who have experienced an initial hypersensitivity reaction to paclitaxel can be safely retreated without further problems. Any attempt to retreat a patient must weigh the relative benefit of treatment for that individual patient against the risk of a severe hypersensitivity reaction. The majority of paclitaxel reactions will be histamine-release reactions (flushing, urticaria, and chest tightness), which resolve with discontinuation of the medication and readministration of dexamethasone (or hydrocortisone) and diphenhydramine. Infu-

▬ Table 9.2
Treatment of Acute Allergic Reactions

Symptom	Therapy	Dosage
Hives Flushing	Diphenhydramine	25 mg i.v. × 1, may repeat × 1
	Cimetidine (or ranitidine)	300 mg (or 50 mg of ranitidine) i.v. × 1
	Normal saline	500-mL bolus × 1
Shortness of breath Wheezing	Diphenhydramine Albuterol	50 mg i.v. × 1 2.5 mg/3 mL of saline via nebulizer × 1.
Chest tightness	Hydrocortisone	100 mg i.v. × 1
	Cimetidine (or ranitidine)	300 mg (or 50 mg of ranitidine) i.v. × 1
	Epinephrine	0.3–0.5 mL of 1:1,000 dilution (0.3–0.5 mg) SQ q10–20 minutes
Stridor Severe bronchospasm Hypoxia Hypotension[a]	Oxygen	Initially 100% via face mask
	Epinephrine	0.3–0.5 mL of 1:1,000 dilution (0.3–0.5 mg) SQ q10–20 minutes
	Normal saline	500-mL bolus × 1
	Hydrocortisone	100 mg i.v. × 1
	Diphenhydramine	50 mg i.v. × 1
	Cimetidine (or ranitidine)	300 mg (or 50 mg of ranitidine) i.v. × 1

[a] Hypotension may require an epinephrine drip (1 mL of 1:1,000 dilution in 500 mL of D5W i.v. at 1 μg/min and titrate to effect) or norepinephrine drip (1–30 μg/min i.v.).

sions can usually be restarted after 15 to 20 minutes without complication.

Some clinicians will retreat a patient following a hypersensitivity reaction to paclitaxel by administering dexamethasone (20 mg) or hydrocortisone (100mg) i.v. every 6 hours for 24 hours before retreatment. The decision to retreat a patient must be individualized, based on each patient's history and prognosis. Patients who have had severe bronchospastic reactions, hypotension, or laryngeal edema should not be rechallenged.

■■■ Extravasation of Irritant and Vesicant Agents

■■■ Pathophysiology

An irritant is an agent that produces a local venous response with or without a skin reaction. Symptoms may include tenderness or burning along the vein with local erythema. These symptoms are usually short lasting and do not result in tissue damage. In contrast, a vesicant is an agent capable of producing extensive tissue damage, with ulceration and necrosis, if extravasated into the surrounding tissue. Some drugs used in the treatment of gynecologic malignancies that are capable of producing extravasation injuries include doxorubicin, dactinomycin, mitomycin, vincristine, and etoposide. Leakage of these agents into the subcutaneous tissue can result in local tissue necrosis, which heals only with great difficulty. Resulting ulcer formation tends to heal very poorly and may result in extended disability. The mechanism of necrosis appears to be tight binding of the drug to the subcutaneous tissue, causing local injury and subsequent cell death. The process repeats itself when the drug is released from the dead cells and thus is available to bind to the next tissue layer.

■■■ Management

The best approach to management of extravasation injury appears to be prevention by administering the agent through a freely flowing intravenous line or indwelling central venous catheter. Individuals administering the drug must be properly trained in techniques of intravenous access and aware of the early signs and symptoms of extravasation including discomfort, burning, and erythema. Slowing of i.v. flow and leakage at the needle insertion site are other signs of extravasation. Pain, edema, induration, and ulceration occur later. Careful attention must be given to selecting the site for drug administration. Large veins are preferable avoiding those over joints or in the antecubital region. Veins of the forearm are preferred, while veins distal to a recent site of access or attempted access should be avoided for at least 24 hours. After obtaining venous access, maintenance fluid should be administered through the line to ensure patency. Before administration of the vesicant, the line should be gently flushed with 5 to 10 mL of normal saline. The vesicant can then be slowly infused at a rate of 1 or 2 mL per minute, while close attention is paid to any patient complaints.

In the event of extravasation, drug infusion must be discontinued immediately, and an attempt to withdraw any remaining drug in the line should be made, as the severity of the reaction depends on the drug and its concentration. Flushing the line with saline can further dilute the drug. If extravasation occurs at a peripheral site, the extremity should be elevated to decrease swelling. Along with the administration of hot or cold compresses, depending on the drug, various antidotes can be administered around the site of infiltration (Table 9.3). If pain, erythema, or swelling persists, a plastic surgery consult should be obtained in the event that the patient may require debridement.

■■■ *Mucositis*

■■■ Pathophysiology

Approximately 40% of patients receiving primary chemotherapy will develop oral complications with each cycle of treatment, due to the toxic effect of the drug on the oral mucosa or to myelosuppression. Patients with hematologic malignancies are at greater risk than those with solid tumors, as are younger patients and those with poor oral hygiene. Drugs used in the treatment of gynecologic malignancies that are associated with mucositis include methotrexate, fluorouracil,

Table 9.3
Antidotes for Vesicant Drugs

Drug	Antidote	Preparation	Administration	Compress
Doxorubicin	Dimethylsulfoxide	50–99% (wt/vol) solution	Apply 1.5 mL topically and allow to air dry; repeat every 4–6 hours for 3–14 days	Cold (inhibits cytotoxicity; heat worsens toxicity)
Cisplatin[a]	Sodium thiosulfate	10% sodium thiosulfate	Use 2 mL for each 100 mg of cisplatin; inject subcutaneously	Cold
Dactinomycin Mitomycin C	None proven Dimethylsulfoxide	50–99% (wt/vol) solution	Apply 1.5 mL topically and allow to air dry; repeat every 4–6 hours for 3–14 days	Cold Cold
Paclitaxel	Hyaluronidase	Wydase—150 U/mL	Inject 1–6 mL (150–900 U) SQ into extravasated site with multiple injections; repeat dosing SQ over next several hours	Cold
Vincristine, etoposide	Hyaluronidase	Wydase—150 U/mL	Inject 1–6 mL (150–900 U) SQ into extravasated site with multiple injections; repeat dosing SQ over next several hours *Action:* Enhances absorption and dispersion of extravasated drug	Warm (increases systemic absorption; cold worsens toxicity)

[a]Vesicant potential with a concentration of more than 20 mL of 0.5-mg/mL extravasates.

dactinomycin, doxorubicin, mitomycin, vincristine, and hydroxyurea.

Drug-induced mucositis is related to the rapid 7- to 14-day turnover of cells lining the oral mucosa. Chemotherapy causes a decrease in the renewal rate of the basal epithelium, resulting in mucosal atrophy and, eventually, ulceration. Decreased nutritional intake exacerbates the problem by depriving the cells of needed nutrients. The most commonly affected areas include the buccal, labial, and soft palate mucosa, as well as the ventral surface of the tongue and the floor of the mouth. Mucositis is generally observed 5 to 7 days following drug administration and tends to resolve within 2 or 3 weeks if left untreated.

■■■■ Management

The major morbidity incurred from mucositis is pain and the resultant inability to eat. Routine and systemic oral care may reduce the degree of mucositis and any subsequent infectious complications. Treatment is directed toward providing symptomatic relief. A 15-mL solution of 2% viscous lidocaine can be used as a 30-second rinse every 3 hours for pain relief, with systemic pain medication added as needed. A 50/50 mix of diphenhydramine and attapulgite (Kaopectate) is an effective rinse that can be used every 2 or 3 hours to provide relief by coating the mucosa. Patients are often unable to eat, but usually find that ice chips and cold drinks provide some relief. Milk of magnesia (MOM) rinses should be avoided, as MOM is a desiccant. If mucositis is accompanied by oropharyngeal *Candida* infection, oral antifungal agents, such as nystatin or miconazole, can be used.

■■■■ *Neurotoxicity*

■■■■ Pathophysiology

Neurotoxicity is the dose-limiting toxicity of one of the most important chemotherapeutic agents used in the treatment of gynecologic cancer, cisplatin.

Cisplatin-induced neuropathy can be manifested as peripheral sensory neuropathy, autonomic dysfunction, ototoxicity, retinal toxicity, and seizures. The incidence of cisplatin neurotoxicity ranges from 15% to 85%, depending on cumulative dose, duration of treatment, concomitant use of other neurotoxic drugs, and underlying medical conditions.

Peripheral neuropathy is the most common form of cisplatin neurotoxicity. Symptoms include paresthesias involving the feet, legs, hands, and arms. Classically, this is described as a stocking/glove distribution. Eventually, there is a loss of deep tendon reflexes and vibratory sensation. This can ultimately lead to difficulty in walking and the ability to perform fine motor movements. The pathophysiology of platinum-induced neuropathy is thought to be related to the accumulation of inorganic platinum within the dorsal root ganglia.

Paclitaxel can cause a similar neurotoxicity to that of cisplatin in up to 25% of patients, especially if underlying medical conditions exist, such as diabetic or alcoholic neuropathy. This may be exacerbated by concomitant administration with cisplatin, because the two have different mechanisms of neurotoxicity. The mechanism of paclitaxel neurotoxicity probably involves the microtubules of both motor and sensory nerve axons. Paclitaxel stabilizes and alters the functioning of these neuronal microtubules, which are critical to the survival and health of the axon. The first symptoms are usually seen in the axons that stretch out the longest from the spinal cord to the toes and hands, but fine sensory nerves can also be affected.

■■■ Management

Treatment of cisplatin neurotoxicity involves discontinuation of the drug. Symptoms may progress for a period after discontinuation of the drug, only to improve several months later. Improvement can continue even 1 or 2 years after discontinuing treatment. Because the treatment of neurotoxicity is limited, preventive agents have been investigated. Amifostine is a prodrug that is converted to a free-radical scavenger and may exhibit a protective effect against cisplatin neurotoxicity. Carboplatin has lower nonhematologic toxicity and has replaced cisplatin when administered in combination with paclitaxel.

▬▬ *Palmar-Plantar Erythrodysesthesia Syndrome (Hand-foot Syndrome)*

▬▬ Pathophysiology

This syndrome is characterized by a cutaneous reaction of the skin on the soles of the feet and palms of the hands. The patients develop erythematous plaques on their hands and feet that can become extremely painful and can lead to cracking of the skin. Patients may initially complain of tingling sensations in their hands and feet that generally progress to swelling, pain, tenderness to touch, intense erythema with blanching between joints, and eventually desquamation. This adverse effect has been reported to occur in patients being treated with liposomal doxorubicin in as many as one third of cases. Other agents that may cause similar symptoms are fluorouracil, docetaxel, and vinorelbine. The symptoms most likely result from a direct dermatologic toxicity from the prolonged blood levels of this cytotoxic agent, and may last several weeks.

▬▬ Management

Treatment of this syndrome is focused on pain relief (systemic and local measures), elevation of the extremities, and prevention of superinfection. Various salves have been used to treat this adverse effect. Pyridoxine and topical dimethylsulfoxide have also been suggested remedies. In severe cases, dose modification or discontinuation of therapy may be indicated.

Selected Reading

Albanell J, Baselga J: Systemic therapy emergencies. *Semin Oncol* 2000; 27:347–361.

Brown KA, Esper P, Kelleher LO, (eds) et al: *Chemotherapy and Biotherapy Guidelines and Recommendations for Practice.* Oncology Nursing Society Publishing Division, Pittsburgh, 2001, pp. 60–62.

Cadman E: Toxicity of chemotherapeutic agents. In FF Becker (ed.), *Cancer: A Comprehensive Treatise,* vol. 5. Plenum Publishing, New York, 1977, p. 59.

Cancer Chemotherapy Guidelines. *Recommendations for the Management of Vesicant Extravasation, Hypersensitivity, and Anaphylaxis.* Oncology Nursing Society, 1999.

Clamon GH: Extravasation. In MC Perry (ed.) *The Chemotherapy Source Book,* 3rd edition. Lippincott Williams & Wilkins, Philadelphia, 2001, p. 432.

Cleri LB, Haywood R: *Oncology Pocket Guide to Chemotherapy,* 5th edition. Mosby, Philadelphia, 2002, pp. 1–20.

Dunton CJ: Management of treatment-related toxicity in advanced ovarian cancer. *Oncologist* 2002; 7(suppl 5):11–19.

Fischer DS, Tish Knobf M, Durivage HJ: *The Cancer Chemotherapy Handbook.* Mosby, St. Louis, 1997, pp. 452–475.

Rowinsky EK, Cazenave LA, Donehower RC: Taxol: A novel investigational antimicrotubule agent. *J Natl Cancer Inst* 1990; 82:1247–1259.

Thomson MICROMEDEX database: MICROMEDEX(R) Healthcare Series Vol. 116. Expires June 2003.

Wiernik PH, Schwartz EL, Strauman JJ, et al: Phase I clinical and pharmacokinetics study of Taxol. *Cancer Res* 1987; 47:2486.

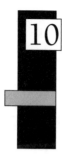

10

USE OF BLOOD PRODUCTS AND HEMATOLOGIC GROWTH FACTORS

MARK A. MORGAN

Red Cells

Indications

Blood component therapy, rather than whole blood, is used in most instances today because it allows specific treatment of deficits and it helps to conserve blood resources (Table 10.1). Red blood cells (RBCs), platelets, and cryoprecipitate or fresh-frozen plasma can be obtained from a single unit of whole blood.

A unit of whole blood consists of approximately 450 mL, and the RBCs are viable for up to 6 weeks when refrigerated. Whole blood is not a reliable source of platelets, granulocytes, or the labile coagulation factors V and VIII. Whole blood is often reserved for catastrophic hemorrhage to simultaneously restore oxygen-carrying capacity, volume, and coagulation factors. This end result, however, can often be achieved using component therapy in addition to crystalloid or colloid solutions.

Packed RBCs can be prepared by centrifuging whole blood and removing the plasma or by apheresis. The red cells are concentrated to a hematocrit of approximately 60% to 75% and a volume of about 200 ml. They are usually refrigerated and citrate-phosphate dextrose (CPD) or CPD adenine-1 are used as preservatives. The shelf life is approximately 42 days.

Chemotherapy of Gynecologic Cancers: Society of Gynecologic Oncologists Handbook 2e, edited by Stephen C. Rubin, MD, Lippincott Williams & Wilkins, Philadelphia © 2004.

▪▪ Table 10.1
Characteristics of Commonly Used Blood Products

Blood Product	Volume (mL)	Hepatitis/ HIV Risk	CMV[a] Risk	Storage Time
Whole blood	450	+	+	35 days
Packed RBCs	200	+	+	42 days
Platelets	50	+	+	5 days[b]
Granulocytes	220	+	+++	24 hours
Fresh-frozen plasma	250	+	0	1 year
Albumin 25%/5%	50/250	0	0	Dated

[a]Risk of CMV from RBCs and platelets may be reduced by leukocyte-depleting filters. CMV-seronegative donors should be used for immunocompromised patients.
[b]Single donor platelets should be transfused within 24 hours.
CMV, cytomegalovirus; RBCs, red blood cells.

When the blood type is rare, RBCs may be frozen in a glycerol solution for up to 10 years but need to be washed of the glycerol and used within 24 hours of thawing.

Transfusion of RBCs is indicated to increase the oxygen-carrying capacity of anemic patients. Oxygen-carrying capacity is adequate for most patients when the hemoglobin is 7 or 8 g/dL. This level may not be sufficient, however, in patients with chronic lung or cardiovascular disease. When anemia is treatment related (i.e., chemotherapy), it is generally not seen until 60 to 90 days after treatment has begun because the average life span of the existing RBCs is 120 days. In the setting of chemotherapy, transfusion may be indicated in anemic patients who suffer significant fatigue, shortness of breath, tachycardia, or orthostasis. One unit of packed RBCs will increase the hemoglobin by approximately 1 g/dL in a 70-kg woman.

▪▪▪ Administration

Red blood cells must be ABO compatible and crossmatched to confirm compatibility with ABO and other antibodies. All blood products should be carefully checked by two individuals to ensure correct identification. Warming the blood is generally not necessary except in the presence of cold agglutinin disease or with rapid transfusion of multiple units. Filters are used to remove debris. In special circumstances, leukocyte-depleting filters can be used to reduce the incidence of febrile nonhemolytic transfusion reactions and also to lower the risk of cytomegalovirus (CMV) infections, which are carried through the leukocytes. Packed RBCs can be mixed with normal saline to increase the rate at which the transfusion can be given. Calcium-containing solutions such as lactated Ringer's will cause the blood to clot and should not be used with transfusion. In the nonemergent setting, 1 U of RBCs is usually transfused over 1 to 3 hours. In critical situations, uncrossmatched type-specific or type 0–negative blood may be used.

Complications

Approximately 1 in 100,000 U of RBCs transfused will result in a fatal hemolytic reaction, usually from ABO incompatibility. Patients with hemolytic reactions often complain of chest or back pain, pain at the infusion site, and restlessness. They may have high fevers and chills. When these signs and symptoms are present the blood infusion should be stopped immediately and the identity of both donor and recipient should be rechecked. Blood pressure and renal function must be supported. Febrile, nonhemolytic reactions are due to recipient antibodies against leukocyte and platelet antigens. Antihistamines and antipyretics are often adequate; however, leukocyte-reduced components may be necessary.

Blood transfusion can transmit bacterial, viral, and protozoal infection. Hepatitis C was the most common form of transfusion-related hepatitis and more than 50% of infected patients progress to chronic liver disease. However, improvements in antibody techniques and the introduction of nucleic acid amplification testing in 1999 have reduced the risk of hepatitis C and human immunodeficiency virus

(HIV) type 1 infection to less than 1 case per 1 million units transfused (Table 10.2). Cytomegalovirus is transmitted in leukocytes and can be an important pathogen in immuno-suppressed patients. Such patients should receive compo-nents from either seronegative donors or from blood that has had the leukocytes removed or have been irradiated. Bacterial growth in refrigerated specimens is uncommon, al-though malaria and Chagas' disease are causes of transfu-sion-related disease outside of the United States. Although

■■■■ Table 10.2

Current Tests for Infectious Agents in Donated Blood

Hepatitis B surface antigen	Screening became mandatory
Hepatitis B core antibody	in 1972; in 2000, post-transfusion hepatitis B estimated at 1 in 137,000
Hepatitis C virus antibody	Risk of transmission now less than 1 in 1,000,000 transfused units since the addition of NAT
HIV-1 and HIV-2 antibody	Antigen test can detect the virus 1 week earlier than the antibody tests; with NAT, estimated risk is less than 1 in 1,900,000
HTLV-I and HTLV-II antibody	HTLV-II is endemic in the Americas and infrequently causes neurologic disease or increased susceptibility to infection
Serologic test for syphilis	Instituted after WWII; no case of transfusion related transmission for many years
Nucleic acid amplification testing	Detects genetic material of HCV and HIV; allows for earliest detection

HCV, hepatitis C virus; HIV; human immunodeficiency virus; HTLV, human T-cell lymphotrophic virus; NAT, nucleic acid amplification testing.

there has never been a documented case of Creutzfeldt-Jakob disease or variant Creutzfeldt-Jakob (mad cow) disease transmitted through the blood, the American Red Cross now defers donors if they have lived in the United Kingdom for a total of 3 months since 1980, any combination of other European countries for 6 months since 1980, or who have received a blood transfusion in the United Kingdom since 1980. Recent documented cases of transmission of West Nile virus in blood has lead to the development of a nucleic acid test which will be undergoing clinical trials in the near future. To date, there have been no documented cases of transmission of the virus responsible for severe acute respiratory syndrome (SARS). Donors are being excluded if they have been exposed to someone with SARS or have recently traveled to a SARS-endemic area of the world.

The average unit of RBCs contains 10 to 20 mEq of potassium and hyperkalemia is a risk in patients with renal compromise who receive multiple units. Circulatory overload may occur in patients with cardiovascular disease. Citrate toxicity, manifested primarily by hypocalcemia, can occur after multiple transfusions, as can iron overload.

▬▬ Platelets

▬▬ Indications

Platelet concentrates (RDP) are usually prepared by centrifugation of platelet-rich plasma from 4 to 8 U of random donor blood. Alternatively, single-donor platelets (SDP) can be prepared by apheresis to yield approximately the same amount of platelets. The total volume is usually about 50 mL, which is stored at room temperature in gas-permeable containers. The platelets remain viable for up to 5 days.

Platelet transfusions are indicated in the presence of severe thrombocytopenia or platelet dysfunction when there is active bleeding or a high risk of bleeding. The risk of spontaneous bleeding increases as the platelet count drops below 20,000/mm^3. Platelet transfusion is most often used in the patient on chemotherapy to maintain the platelet count greater than 10,000 to 20,000. Recent evidence suggests that counts as low as 5,000 to 10,000 may be safe. Bleeding complications are more common with platelet counts this low, but are not usually severe. The platelet count threshold for transfusion should be higher in the presence of sepsis, bleeding, or a rapidly decreasing platelet count.

Prophylactic transfusion before abdominal surgery is usually not required until counts are less than 50,000/mm^3 in the absence of other risk factors for bleeding. Platelets should not be given routinely for massive transfusion, but used in the presence of microvascular bleeding when counts are less than 100,000/mm^3.

████ Administration

Platelet concentrates are infused through a standard blood bank filter over 10 to 20 minutes. One unit of RDP should increase the platelet count by 5,000 to 10,000 platelets/mm^3. A unit of SDP should increase the platelet count by 30,000 to 40,000/mm^3.

A platelet count should be obtained at 1 and 24 hours after transfusion. Alloimmunization would be manifested by a poor 1-hour post-transfusion increment, whereas a poor increment at 24 hours can represent a number of conditions including alloimmunization, bleeding, fever, infection, immunodestruction, hypersplenism, or disseminated intravascular coagulation. Patients with a poor response at 1 hour should receive human leukocyte antigen (HLA)-matched single-donor platelets if subsequent transfusions are needed. Alloimmunization can occur because small amounts of RBCs and leukocytes are present in platelets. For this reason, platelets should also be matched when possible for ABO and Rh type. Leukoreduced platelets should be used in patients expected to receive multiple transfusions.

■■■ Complications

The most frequent complication of platelet transfusion is the development of alloantibodies to the HLA antigens on lymphocytes present in the platelet concentrates. Also, because platelets are stored at room temperature, small amounts of contaminating microorganisms may increase as the storage time increases, resulting in sepsis. Patients occasionally have fever and urticaria, and the risk of viral transmission is the same as for RBCs. Rh sensitization can occur if an Rh-negative woman is given platelets from an Rh-positive donor. Administration of Rh_o immunoglobulin can prevent sensitization.

■■■ *Clotting Factors*

■■■ Indications

Clotting factors are most often replaced by the use of fresh-frozen plasma or cryoprecipitate, or less commonly with specific factor (i.e., factor IX) concentrates. Fresh-frozen plasma (FFP) is separated from whole blood within 6 to 8 hours of collection in a volume of approximately 250 mL. It can be stored for up to 1 year at 18°C. It is indicated in cases of multiple coagulation factor deficiencies, usually in the presence of an elevated prothrombin time or activated partial thromboplastin time. FFP may also be used for emergency reversal of warfarin but should not be used as a volume expander.

Cryoprecipitate or cryoprecipitated antihemophilic factor is prepared from fresh-frozen plasma by cold precipitation. The usual volume is 10 to 25 mL and contains approximately 50% of the fibrinogen, factor VIII:C, factor VIII:vWF (von Willebrand factor), and factor XIII found in the original unit of plasma. It is most commonly used for replacement of factor VIII and XIII deficiencies and for the treatment of von Willebrand's disease if factor VIII concentrate is not available. Recently, recombinant factor VII has become available. This factor has been used in cases of bleeding due to inhibitors to factors VIII and IX as well as platelet disorders and intractable surgical hemorrhage.

■■■ Administration

Fresh-frozen plasma requires 10 to 30 minutes to thaw and is usually given as a 1- or 2-U transfusion in the presence of documented factor deficiency, as manifested by a prothrombin time greater than 1.5 times normal. FFP should be ABO compatible. Cryoprecipitate is also stored in a frozen state and is usually given in a dose of 10 to 20 U in a volume of about 15 mL/U within 6 hours of thawing. ABO compatibility is preferable.

■■■ Complications

Fresh-frozen plasma carries the same risk of viral infection (i.e., hepatitis, HIV) as blood. However, because cryoprecipitate is a pooled product from usually 10 to 20 donors, there is an added risk. Clotting factor concentrates that have been treated to eliminate infectious agents and recombinant proteins are becoming more available and may replace cryoprecipitate. Severe immunological reactions have been reported due to antibodies present in plasma.

■■■ *Granulocytes*

■■■ Indications

In patients with solid tumors, the frequency of infection increases as the absolute neutrophil count decreases below 500 cells/mm^3, and infection is the major cause of chemotherapy-related mortality in these patients. Severe and prolonged neutropenia is becoming less common with the use of recombinant myeloid growth factors, and the indications for granulocyte transfusions have become less common. However, certain patients with sepsis unresponsive to antibiotic therapy for 48 hours and an expected du-

ration of severe neutropenia for 1 week or more may benefit from granulocyte transfusion. This generally refers to
bacterial sepsis, because the role for granulocyte transfusion
in fungal sepsis is unclear. Prophylactic granulocyte transfusion is not indicated.

Granulocytes are usually obtained by the use of a contin-
uous-flow cell separator. A low-molecular-weight starch is
used to aid in the separation of granulocytes, and donors
may be pretreated with either steroids or granulocyte
colony-stimulating factors (G-CSF) to increase the yield.

▬▬ Administration

Granulocytes are stored at 22°C and they begin to lose
their function after 24 to 48 hours. Usually, they are transfused within a few hours of apheresis but must be transfused within 24 hours. Granulocytes should be transfused
daily until either the granulocyte count recovers or the patient is afebrile and off antibiotics for 2 or 3 days. Patients
with evidence of alloimmunization should receive HLA-
matched granulocytes or have leukocyte crossmatching.
Greater than 10^{10} cells per transfusion should be given
daily, as the normal granulocyte production is approximately 10^{11} cells per day.

▬▬ Complications

Granulocyte transfusions carry the same risk of viral transmission for both hepatitis and HIV as RBCs, but they also
carry a significant risk for CMV infection. Therefore, CMV-
seropositive donors should not be used for a CMV-seronegative recipient. In addition, because granulocytes have HLA
antigens and granulocyte-specific antigens on their surface,
alloimmunization is common. This can cause chills and
fever in their recipient. Pulmonary toxicity has also been reported, although this is significantly less when a cell separator is used for obtaining the granulocytes, as opposed to the
older method of leukofiltration. Graft versus host disease is

also possible in a severely immunocompromised host because there are significant amounts of lymphocytes in the granulocyte transfusion. This can be eliminated by irradiation before transfusion.

■■■ *Granulocyte Colony-stimulating Factor*

■■■ Indications

Commercially available G-CSF is a glycoprotein produced by recombinant DNA technology that stimulates the proliferation and differentiation of the relatively mature granulocyte progenitor. It also may enhance granulocyte survival and affect the function and migration of mature neutrophils. Granulocyte-macrophage colony-stimulating factor (GM-CSF) is also available in the United States but is used less often, presumably because of the increased incidence of fever, flu-like symptoms, hypotension, pleuritis, and pericarditis, which is thought to be secondary to monocyte activation and elaboration of proinflammatory cytokines.

G-CSF is indicated to decrease the incidence of febrile neutropenia in patients receiving chemotherapy for non-myeloid malignancies with regimens associated with a significant incidence (e.g., 40% or higher) of neutropenia with fever. It is unclear whether the level of dose escalation permitted by the use of these growth factors will improve survival. They should not be used routinely in neutropenic patients who are afebrile. It is not recommended for the routine treatment of febrile neutropenia.

Both G-CSF and GM-CSF can elaborate bone marrow progenitor cells into the peripheral blood where they can be harvested and then transplanted in support of dose-intensive chemotherapy. G-CSF may also be useful in established febrile neutropenia in certain high-risk patients when granulocyte recovery is expected to be prolonged. G-CSF may be considered in special circumstances, such as in the presence of an open wound, decreased immune function, or in patients with a history of extensive chemotherapy or pelvic radiotherapy. It is not recommended in patients receiving concomitant chemotherapy and radiotherapy.

■■■ Administration

The recommended dosage of G-CSF (filgrastim) is 5 µg/kg/day by subcutaneous injection. Dosages of 10 µg/kg/day or higher have been used in clinical trials and may prove beneficial. Intravenous administration is not as effective, but may be used in special circumstances. Therapy should begin at least 24 hours after completion of chemotherapy and continue daily until the expected nadir is past and the neutrophil count is about 10,000/mm^3. It is expected there will be about a 50% drop in the neutrophil count within 48 hours of discontinuing the G-CSF The next course of chemotherapy should not begin until at least 48 hours after the last dose of G-CSF, if at all possible. A complete blood count should be obtained before therapy and twice weekly during treatment.

A long-acting version of G-CSF (pegfilgrastim) is now available. It is administered once per chemotherapy cycle in nonmyeloid malignancies. A subcutaneous dose of 6 mg is recommended at least 24 hours after chemotherapy administration and should not be given with 14 days of the next chemotherapy dose.

■■■ Complications

Medullary bone pain is the most common side effect of G-CSF, especially at higher doses. Inflammatory-mediated side effects associated with GM-CSF are usually not seen with G-CSF, although exacerbation of preexisting skin disorders such as psoriasis has been reported, Thrombosis has been reported but may be due to other factors. Mild alopecia and splenomegaly can occur with long-term administration of G-CSF. Decreases in platelet counts have also been observed, as well as minor elevations in lactate dehydrogenase, alkaline phosphatase, and uric acid. The potential for G-CSF to act as a growth factor for myeloid or nonmyeloid malignancies is not certain.

■■■ Erythropoietin

■■■ Indications

Erythropoietin is a hormone produced by the kidney and liver that regulates erythropoiesis. The gene for erythropoietin was cloned in 1985 and subsequently trials in patients with end-stage renal disease showed that recombinant human erythropoietin (rHuEpo) was effective in alleviating the anemia associated with renal insufficiency. Subsequent studies in anemic patients with AIDS or rheumatoid arthritis and in cancer patients undergoing chemotherapy have demonstrated a benefit to treatment with rHuEpo or epoetin. Patients with cancer who are undergoing chemotherapy are often anemic, and there is evidence that cancer patients show an inadequate erythropoietin response to anemia. Epoetin reduces the transfusion requirement in anemic patients and probably enhances the overall quality of life. It is unclear whether epoetin is beneficial in patients with cancer who are not undergoing chemotherapy. Although epoetin administration has also been suggested as an adjunct to radiation therapy, there is no conclusive evidence at present that epoetin improves survival in patients undergoing radiation therapy or chemotherapy.

Epoetin is indicated when there is a significant chance that blood transfusion may be required or the hemoglobin has decreased to concentrations of 10 mg/dL or less during chemotherapy. Defining the proper patients for therapy may be difficult, but patients who start with low hemoglobin concentrations or who have a rapid decrease in hemoglobin concentration with their first course of chemotherapy will most likely need blood. Epoetin is not indicated for the treatment of anemia due to established deficiencies, such as iron or folate. It is important to correct other causes of anemia (especially iron deficiency) before using epoetin. Currently, there is insufficient evidence to support maintaining hemoglobin levels above 12 mg/dL.

▰▰▰ Administration

Epoetin is injected subcutaneously at a dosage of 150 U/kg three times a week for a minimum of 4 weeks; the dosage may be escalated to 300 U/kg three times per week for non-responders. It takes at least 2 weeks to see a clinical effect after beginning epoetin. A less-studied but apparently equivalent approach is to use 40,000 U per week and escalate to 60,000 U for nonresponders. A long-acting erythropoietic agent, darbepoetin alfa, is available. When given at a dosage of 3.0 μg/kg every 3 weeks, darbepoetin alfa produces hematologic effects equivalent to epoetin at 40,000 U/wk. Early results suggest that a fixed dosage of 200 μg of darbepoetin alfa every 2 weeks may also be equivalent.

▰▰▰ Complications

Although worsening of hypertension has been seen in patients with end-stage renal disease, hypertension has not been a problem in other patient populations. Other side effects are rare and minor, such as edema and diarrhea. There is no evidence of a growth factor effect on tumor cells and antibodies to epoetin have not been observed.

▰▰▰ *Oprelvekin*

▰▰▰ Indications

Oprelvekin is a protein produced in *Escherichia coli* by recombinant DNA methods. The protein differs from native interleukin-11 (IL-11) only in lacking the amino-terminal proline residue. IL-11 stimulates the proliferation and maturation of megakaryocyte progenitor cells, resulting in increased platelet production. There is no measurable difference in bioactivity either *in vitro* or *in vivo* between IL-11 and oprelvekin. Oprelvekin is indicated for the prevention of severe thrombocytopenia in adult patients on chemotherapy for nonmyeloid malignancies.

▬ Administration

Oprelvekin is injected subcutaneously 6 to 24 hours after chemotherapy administration at a dosage of 50 μg/kg daily for 10 to 21 days. It should be continued until the postnadir platelet count is at least 50,000 per microliter. It should be discontinued at least 2 days before the next chemotherapy dose.

▬ Complications

Oprelvekin has been associated with fluid retention resulting in generalized edema, pulmonary edema, hemodilution, electrolyte abnormalities and arrhythmias. Anaphylaxis has also been reported.

Selected Reading

Cable R, Carlson B, Chambers K, et al: Practice guidelines for blood transfusion: A compilation from recent peer-reviewed literature. *Am Natl Red Cross* 2002.

College of American Pathologists: Practice parameter for the use of fresh-frozen plasma, cryoprecipitate, and platelets. *JAMA* 1994; 271:777–781.

Miller LL (ed.): American Society of Clinical Oncology recommendations for the use of hematopoietic colony-stimulating factors: Evidence-based, clinical practice guidelines. *J Clin Oncol* 1994; 12:2471–2508.

Ozer H, Armitage JO, Bennett CL, et al: Update of recommendations for the use of hematopoietic colony stimulating factors: Evidence based clinical practice guidelines. *J Clin Oncol* 2000; 18:3558–3585.

Rizzo D, Lichtin AE, Woolf SH, et al: Use of epoetin in patients with cancer: Evidence-based clinical practice guidelines of the American Society of Clinical Oncology an the American Society of Hematology. *J Clin Oncol* 2002; 20:4083–4107.

Rubenstein EB, Elting L: Incorporating new modalities into practice guidelines: platelet growth factors. *Oncology* 1998; 12(11A):381–386.

Schiffer CA: Granulocyte transfusion: An overlooked therapeutic modality. *Transfus Med Rev* 1990; 4:2.

Stehling L, Simon TL: The red blood cell transfusion trigger. Physiology and clinical studies. *Arch Pathol Lab Med* 1994; 118:429–434.

Simon TL, Alverson DC, AuBuchon J, et al: Practice parameter for the use of red blood cell transfusions: Developed by the Red Blood Cell Administration Practice Guidelines Development Task Force of the College of American Pathologists. *Arch Pathol Lab Med* 1998; 122:130–138.

Schiffer CA, Anderson KC, Bennett CL, et al: Platelet transfusion for patients with cancer: Clinical practice guidelines of the American Society of Clinical Oncology. *J Clin Oncol* 2001; 19:1519–1538.

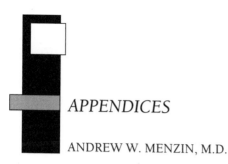

APPENDICES

ANDREW W. MENZIN, M.D.

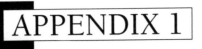

APPENDIX 1

DEFINITIONS OF RESPONSE

COMPLETE RESPONSE (CR): Complete resolution of all evidence of disease lasting at least 1 month

- Complete Clinical Response (CCR)
- Complete Pathologic Response (CPR): surgically documented

PARTIAL RESPONSE (PR): A decrease of greater than or equal to 50% in the product of the diameters (maximal and minimal) of all measurable lesions lasting at least 1 month without the development of new lesions

- Partial Clinical Response (PCR)
- Partial Pathologic Response (PPR): surgically documented

STABLE DISEASE (SD): A decrease of less than 50% or an increase of less than 25% in the product of the diameters of all measurable lesions

PROGRESSION: An increase of greater than or equal to 25% in the measurable lesions as described above or the identification of new lesions

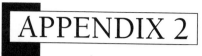

APPENDIX 2

PERFORMANCE STATUS

GOG* Score	ECOG** Score	Karnofsky Score	Activity Level
0	0	90–100	Fully active, unrestricted activities of daily living.
1	1	70–80	Ambulatory, but restricted in strenuous activity.
2	2	50–60	Ambulatory, but capable of self-care. Unable to work. Out of bed greater than 50% of waking hours.
3	3	30–40	Limited self-care, or confined to bed or chair 50% of waking hours, needs special assistance.
4	4	10–20	Completely disabled, and no self-care.
5	5	0	Dead.

*GOG = Gynecologic Oncology Group.
**ECOG = Eastern Cooperative Oncology Group.

APPENDIX 3 *GOG Common Toxicity Criteria*

				Grade		
	Toxicity	**0**	**1**	**2**	**3**	**4**
Blood/Bone	WBC	≥4.0	3.0–3.9	2.0–2.9	1.0–1.9	<1.0
Marrow	PLT	WNL	75.0–normal	50.0–74.9	25.0–49.9	<25.0
	Hgb	WNL	10.0–normal	8.0–10.0	6.5–7.9	<6.5
	Granulocytes/Bands	≥2.0	1.5–1.9	1.0–1.4	0.5–0.9	<0.5
	Lymphocytes	≥2.0	1.5–1.9	1.0–1.4	0.5–0.9	<0.5
	Hemorrhage (clinical including operative)	None	Mild, no transfusion	Gross, 1–2 units transfusion per episode	Gross, 3–4 units transfusion per episode	Massive >4 units transfusion per episode
	Infection	None	Mild	Moderate	Severe	Life-threatening
GI	Nausea	None	Able to eat Reasonable intake	Intake significantly decreased but can eat	No significant intake	—
	Vomiting	None	1 episode in 24 hr	2–5 episodes in 24 hr	6–10 episodes in 24 hr	>10 episodes in 24 hr or requiring parenteral support
	Diarrhea	None	Increase of 2–3 stools/day over pre-Rx	Increase of 4–6 stools/day, or nocturnal stools, or moderate cramping	Increase of 7–9 stools/day, or incontinence or severe cramping	Increase of 10 stools/day or grossly bloody diarrhea or need for parenteral support

Stomatitis	None	Painless erythema, edema, or ulcers, or mild soreness	Painful erythema, edema, or ulcers, but can eat	Painful erythema, edema, or ulcers, and cannot eat	Requires parenteral or enteral support
Mechanical problems	None	Temporary ileus of 3 days or less duration	Ileus requiring tube compression; narrowing of intestinal segment on x-ray or moderate mucosal edema on proctoscopy	Surgically correctable defect, no stoma	Fistula, perforation, chronic bleeding requiring diversion
Operative	None	Repair of mucosal disruption	Resection for enterotomy	Temporary diversion	Permanent diversion
Liver					
Bilirubin	WNL	—	$<1.5 \times N$	$1.6\text{–}3.0 \times N$	$>3.0 \times N$
Transaminase (SGOT, SGPT)	WNL	$\leq 2.5 \times N$	$2.6\text{–}5.0 \times N$	$5.1\text{–}20.0 \times N$	$>20.0 \times N$
Alk. phos. or 5-nucleotidase	WNL	$\leq 2.5 \times N$	$2.6\text{–}5.0 \times N$	$5.1\text{–}20.0 \times N$	$>20.0 \times N$
Liver (clinical)	No change from baseline	—	—	Precoma	Hepatic coma
Kidney/Bladder					
Creatinine	WNL	$<1.5 \times N$	$1.5\text{–}3.0 \times N$	$3.1\text{–}6.0 \times N$	$>6.0 \times N$
Proteinuria	No change	1+ or <0.3 g% or <3 g/l	2-3+ or 0.3–1.0 g% or 3–10 g/l	4+ or >1.0 g% or >10 g/l	Nephrotic syndrome

(continued)

■ APPENDIX 3 GOG Common Toxicity Criteria (continued)

Toxicity	0	1	Grade 2	3	4
Kidney/ Bladder (cont.)					
Hematuria Bladder and ureter, acute	Negative No problems	Micro only Dysuria; frequency and/or microscopic hematuria; injury of bladder with primary repair	Gross, no clots Bacterial infection, gross hematuria not requiring transfusion (<2 g% ↓ in HGB); sepsis, fistula, or obstruction requiring secondary operation; loss of one kidney	Gross and clots Gross hematuria requiring transfusion (>2 g% ↓ in HGB); sepsis, fistula, or obstruction requiring secondary operation; loss of one kidney	Requires transfusion Life-threatening hematuria or septic obstruction of both kidneys or vesicovaginal fistula requiring diversion
Chronic	None	Dysuria; frequency; minimal telangiectasia with edema (cystoscopy)	Superficial ulceration; moderate telangiectasia; gross hematuria (<2 g% ↓ in HGB); bladder volume less than 150 cc	Deep ulceration, severe pain; gross hematuria requiring transfusion (>2 g% ↓ in HGB); permanent unilateral loss of kidney	Decreased bladder volume requiring diversion or catheter drainage; fistula; necrosis; permanent bilateral obstruction or loss of renal function requiring dialysis

Operative	None	Bladder atony immediately postoperative	Bladder atony >6 weeks but transient	Bladder atony requiring intermittent catheterization	—
Alopecia	No loss	Mild hair loss	Pronounced or total hair loss	—	—
Pulmonary	None or no change	Asymptomatic, with abnormality in PFTs	Dyspnea on significant exertion	Dyspnea at normal level of activity	Dyspnea at rest
Heart					
Cardiac-dysrhythmias	None	Asymptomatic, transient, requiring no therapy	Recurrent or persistent, no therapy required	Requires treatment	Requires monitoring, or hypotension, or ventricular tachycardia, or fibrilation
Cardiac-function	None	Asymptomatic, decline of resting ejection fraction by less than 20% of baseline value	Asymptomatic, decline of resting ejection fraction by more than 20% of baseline value	Mild CHF responsive to therapy	Severe or refractory CHF
Cardiac-ischemia	None	Nonspecific T-wave flattening	Asymptomatic, ST and T-wave changes suggesting ischemia	Angina without evidence for infarction	Acute myocardial infarction
Cardiac-pericardial	None	Asymptomatic effusion, no intervention required	Pericarditis (rub, chest pain, ECG changes)	Symptomatic effusion; drainage required	Tamponade; drainage urgently required

(continued)

APPENDIX 3 *GOG Common Toxicity Criteria (continued)*

	Toxicity	0	1	2	3	4
				Grade		
Blood Pressure	Hypertension	None or no change	Asymptomatic, transient increase by greater than 20 mmHg (D) or to >150/100 if previously WNL. No treatment required	Recurrent or persistent increase by greater than 20 mmHg (D) or to >150/100 if previously WNL. No treatment required	Requires therapy	Hypertensive crisis
	Hypotension	None or no change	Changes requiring no therapy (including transient orthostatic hypotension)	Requires fluid replacement or other therapy but not hospitalization	Requires therapy and hospitalization, resolves within 48 hr of stopping the agent	Requires therapy and hospitalization for >48 hr after stopping the agent
	Venous problems	None	Superficial phlebitis; primary suture repair for injury with grade 0 or 1 blood loss	Ischemia not requiring surgical treatment. Primary suture repair for injury with grade 2 or greater blood loss	Pulmonary embolus; bypass for injury	Pulmonary embolus requiring embolectomy or caval ligation

Arterial problems	None	Spasm, primary suture repair for injury with grade 0 or 1 blood loss	Ischemia not requiring surgical treatment. Primary suture repair for injury with grade 2 or greater blood loss	Vascular thrombosis requiring resection with anastomosis. Vascular occlusion requiring surgery; bypass for injury	Myocardial infarction; resection of organ (bowel, limb, etc.)
Neurologic					
Neurosensory	None or no change	Mild paresthesias, loss of deep tendon reflexes	Mild or moderate objective sensory loss; moderate paresthesias	Severe objective sensory loss or paresthesias that interfere with function	—
Neuromotor	None or no change	Subjective weakness; no objective findings	Mild objective weakness without significant impairment	Objective weakness with impairment	Paralysis
Neurocortical	None	Mild somnolence or agitation	Moderate somnolence or agitation	Severe somnolence, agitation, confusion, disorientation, hallucination	Coma, seizures, toxic psychosis
Neurocerebellar	None	Slight incoordination, dysdiadokinesis	Intention tremor, dysmetria, slurred speech, nystagmus	Locomotor ataxia	Cerebellar necrosis
Neuro-mood	No change	Mild anxiety or depression	Moderate anxiety or depression	Severe anxiety or depression	Suicidal ideation
Neuro-headache	None	Mild	Moderate or severe but transient	Unrelenting and severe	—

(continued)

			Grade		
Toxicity	**0**	**1**	**2**	**3**	**4**
Neurologic (cont.)					
Neuro-constipation	None or no change	Mild	Moderate	Severe	Ileus >96 hr
Neuro-hearing	None or no change	Asymptomatic, hearing loss on audiometry only	Tinnitus	Hearing loss interfering with function but correctable	Deafness not correctable
Neuro-vision	None or no change	—	—	Symptomatic subtotal loss of vision	Blindness
Skin					
Skin	None or no change	Scattered macular or papular eruption or erythema that is asymptomatic	Scattered macular or papular eruption or erythema with pruritus or other associated symptoms	General symptomatic macular, papular, or vesicular eruption	Exfoliative dermatitis or ulcerating dermatitis
Wound-infection	None	Cellulitis	Superficial infection	Abscess	Necrotizing fasciitis
Wound-noninfectious	None	Incisional separation	Incisional hernia	Fascial disruption without evisceration	Fascial disruption with evisceration
Allergy	None	Transient rash, drug fever <38°C (100.4°F)	Urticaria, drug; fever 38°C (100.4°F); mild bronchospasm	Serum sickness, bronchospasm, requiring parenteral meals	Anaphylaxis

	None	37.1–38.0°C (98.7–104.0°F)	38.1–40.0°C (100.5–104.0°F)	>40.0°C (>104.0°F) for less than 24 hr	>40.0°C (104.0°F) for more than 24 hr or fever accompanied by hypotension
Fever in absence of infection	None				
Lymphatics	None	Mild lymphedema	Moderate lymphedema requiring compression; lymphocyst	Severe lymphedema limiting function; lymphocyst requiring surgery	Severe edema limiting function with ulceration
Local	None	Pain	Pain and swelling, with inflammation or phlebitis	Ulceration	Plastic surgery indicated
Metabolic					
Weight gain/loss	<5.0%	5.0–9.9%	10.0–19.9%	>20.0%	—
Hyperglycemia	>116	116–160	161–250	251–500	>500 or ketoacidosis
Hypoglycemia	>64	55–64	40–54	30–39	>30
Amylase	WNL	<1.5 × N	1.5–2.0 × N	2.1–5.0 × N	>5.1 × N
Hypercalcemia	<10.6	10.6–11.5	11.6–12.5	12.6–13.5	>13.5
Hypocalcemia	>8.4	8.4–7.8	7.7–7.0	6.9–6.1	6.0
Hypomagnecemia	>1.4	1.4–1.2	1.1–0.9	0.8–0.6	0.5
Coagulation					
Fibrinogen	WNL	0.99–0.75 × N	0.74–0.50 × N	0.49–0.25 × N	0.24 × N
Prothrombin time	WNL	1.01–1.25 × N	1.26–1.5 × N	1.51–2.00 × N	>2.00 × N
Partial prothrombin time	WNL	1.01–1.66 × N	1.67–2.33 × N	2.34–3.00 × N	>3.00 × N

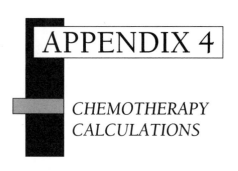

APPENDIX 4

CHEMOTHERAPY CALCULATIONS

Body Surface Area (BSA)

Mostellar equation (m^2): $\sqrt{wt \times ht/3600}$
DuBois and DuBois (m^2): $(wt^{0.425}) \times (ht^{0.725}) \times 71.84$
Haycock (m^2): $(wt^{0.5378}) \times (ht^{0.3964}) \times 0.024265$

m^2 = meters squared
wt = weight in kilograms
ht = height in centimeters

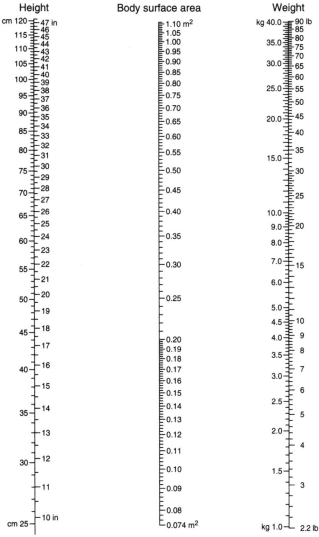

Nomogram for determination of body surface area of children from height and weight. (From Diem K, Lentner C (eds): *Scientific Tables*, ed 7. Basel, Switzerland, Ciba-Geigy, 1962. Used with permission.)

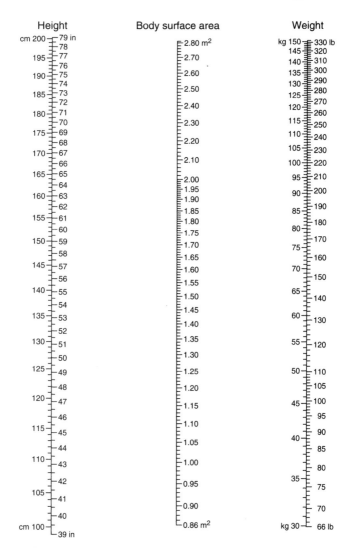

Nomogram for determination of body surface area of adults from
height and weight. (From Diem K, Lentner C (eds): *Scientific Tables*,
ed 7. Basel, Switzerland, Ciba-Geigy, 1962. Used with permission.)

Ideal Body Weight (IBW)*

Males

Ht (cm)	Wt (kg)	Ht (cm)	Wt (kg)	Ht (cm)	Wt (kg)
145	51.9	159	58.9	173	68.7
146	52.4	160	60.5	174	69.4
147	52.9	161	61.1	175	70.1
148	53.6	162	61.7	176	70.8
149	54.0	163	62.3	177	71.6
150	54.5	164	62.9	178	72.4
151	55.0	165	63.5	179	73.3
152	55.8	166	64.0	180	74.2
153	56.1	167	64.6	181	75.0
154	56.6	168	65.2	182	75.6
155	57.2	169	65.9	183	76.5
156	57.9	170	66.6	184	77.3
157	58.6	171	67.3	185	78.1
158	59.3	172	68.0	186	78.9

Females

Ht (cm)	Wt (kg)	Ht (cm)	Wt (kg)	Ht (cm)	Wt (kg)
140	44.9	150	50.4	160	56.2
141	45.4	151	51.0	161	56.9
142	45.9	152	51.5	162	57.6
143	46.4	153	52.0	163	58.3
144	47.0	154	52.5	164	58.9
145	47.5	155	53.1	165	59.5
146	48.0	156	53.7	166	60.1
147	48.6	157	54.3	167	60.7
148	49.2	158	54.9	168	61.4
149	49.8	159	55.5	169	62.1

*Nude weight without shoes.

Creatinine Clearance (CrCl)

Based on a timed urine collection

$$\frac{\text{Urine Creatinine}}{\text{Serum Creatinine}} \times \frac{\text{Urine Volume}}{\text{Time}}$$

Based on age, weight, and serum creatinine

Method of Cockcroft and Gault

$$CrCl_{men} = \frac{(140 - Age) \times (Lean\ Body\ Wt)}{(Serum\ Creatinine) \times 72}$$

$$CrCl_{women} = CrCl_{men} \times 0.85$$

Method of Jeliffe

$$\frac{CrCl}{1.73} = \frac{100}{Serum\ Creatinine} - 2$$

CrCl = ml/min
Time = duration of collection in minutes
Age = years
Weight (Wt) = kg
Urine Volume = ml
Urine Creatinine = mg/dl
Serum Creatinine = mg/dl

Carboplatin Dosing

AREA UNDER THE CURVE (AUC) METHOD [CALVERT FORMULA]
  Dose (mg) = Target AUC (mg/ml × min) × [CrCl (ml/min) + 25]

  Guidelines:
  Untreated Adults Target AUC for Carboplatin alone = 7
  Previously Treated Adults Target AUC for Carboplatin alone = 5
  Target AUC for Carboplatin in combination = 4.5
  CrCl = Creatinine Clearance

PLATLET NADIR METHOD [EGORIN FORMULA]
  Untreated patients:
  Dose (mg/m^2) = 0.091 × (CrCl/BSA) × (PreRx Plt −
                Desired nadir Plt/PreRx Plt × 100) + 86

Previously treated patients
  Dose (mg/m^2) = 0.091 × (CrCl/BSA) × [(PreRx Plt −
                Desired nadir Plt/PreRx Plt × 100) − 17] + 86

m^2 = meters squared
PreRx Plt = pretreatment platelet count

Modified from Calvert AH, Newell DR, Gumbrell, et al.: Carboplatin dosage: Prospective evaluation of a simple formula based on renal function. *J Clin Oncol* 1989 7:1748–1756; and Egorin MJ, Van Echo DA, Olman EA, et al.: Prospective validation of a pharmacologically based dosing scheme for the cis-diamminedichloroplatinum (II) analogue diamminecyclobutanedicarboxylatoplatinum. *Cancer Res* 1985; 45:6502–6506.

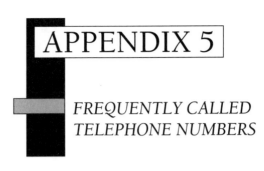

APPENDIX 5

FREQUENTLY CALLED TELEPHONE NUMBERS

SOCIETY OF GYNECOLOGIC ONCOLOGISTS
Administrative Office
(312) 644-6610

GYNECOLOGIC ONCOLOGY GROUP
Administrative Office (protocol, meeting, membership information, etc.)
(800) 225-3053
(215) 854-0770

NATIONAL CANCER INSTITUTE
(800) 4-CANCER
(800) 422-6237

AMERICAN CANCER SOCIETY
National Office
(404) 320-3333
Local Offices
Telephone number in local directories

POISON CONTROL HOTLINE
Telephone number in Emergency section of local directories

ONCOLINK: THE UNIVERSITY OF PENNSYLVANIA CANCER RESOURCE
World-Wide-Web (URL) address:
http://www.oncolink.upenn.edu

APPENDIX 6 *Chemotherapeutic Agents*

Brand Name

Generic Name	USA (Manufacturer)	Europe (Manufacturer)
A. *Antimetabolites*		
5-Fluorouracil (5-FU)	Efudex (Roche)	Efudix (Roche)
	Adrucil (Adria)	Efudex (Hoffman-La Roche)
	Fluoroplex (Allergan)	Adrucil (Pharmacia)
	Ribofluor (Ribosepharm)	
Methotrexate (MTX)	Methotrexate (Lederle)	Matrex (Farmitalia Carlo Erba)
		Metotrexol (Lundbeck)
		Emthexat (Nycomed)
B. *Alkylating Agents*		
Altretamine (HMM)	Hexalen (US Bioscience)	Hexastat (Ballon, Rhone-Poulenc Rorer)
	Hexinawas (Wassermann)	
Carboplatin	Paraplatin (Bristol-Myers Squibb)	Paraplatin (Bristol-Myers Squibb)
		Ribocarbo (Ribopharm)
		Carbosol (Donau-Pharmazie)
Chlorambucil	Leukeran (Burroughs Wellcome)	Leukeran (Burroughs Wellcome)
		Linfolysin (ISM)

(continued)

219

		Brand Name
Generic Name	**USA (Manufacturer)**	**Europe (Manufacturer)**
B. Alkylating Agents (cont.)		
Cisplatin	Platinol (Bristol-Myers Squibb)	Platinol (Bristol-Myers Squibb)
		Platinex (Bristol-Myers Squibb)
		Cismaplat (Bellon)
		Platosin (Conforma)
Cyclophosphamide	Cytoxan (Bristol-Myers Squibb)	Cytoxan (Bristol-Myers Squibb, Pharmachemie)
	Neosan (Adria)	Endoxan (Sarget)
		Procytox (Horner)
		Sendoxan (Pharmacia)
Ifosfamide	Ifex (Bristol-Myers Squibb,	Ifex (Bristol-Myers Squibb)
	Mead Johnson)	Holoxam (Sarget, ASTA Medica)
		Tronoxal (Funk)
Melphalan	Alkeran (Burroughs Wellcome)	Alkeran (Burroughs Wellcome)
Mesna	Mesnex (Bristol-Myers Squibb)	Uromitexan (ASTA Medica,
		Bristol-Myers Squibb, Sarget, Funk)
		Mucofluid (UCB, Bios)
		Mistabron (Diethelm)
		Mistabronco (UCB)

Thiotepa	Thiotepa (Lederle)	Thiotepa (Lederle)
		Oncotiotepa (Simes-Sintesa)
		Ledertepa (Lederle)

C. Antitumor Antibiotics

Bleomycin	Blenoxane (Bristol-Myers Squibb)	Blenoxane (Bristol-Myers Squibb)
		Bleomycinum (Pfizer)
		Bleocin (Krka)
Dactinomycin	Cosmegen (Merck)	Cosmegen (Merck Sharp & Dohme)
Doxorubicin	Rubex (Bristol-Myers Squibb)	Adriblastine (Pharmacia)
	Adriamycin (Adria, Pharmacia)	Adriablastin (Farmasan, Labohain)
	Adriblastina (Chiron)	
Mitomycin C	Mutamycin (Bristol-Myers Squibb)	Mutamycin (Bristol-Myers Squibb)
		Ametycin (Sanofi Winthrop)
		Mito-medac (Medac)
Mitoxantrone	Novantrone (Lederle)	Novantrone (Lederle)

D. Agents Derived from Plants

Etoposide (VP-16)	VePesid (Bristol-Myers Squibb)	VePesid (Bristol-Myers Squibb, Sandoz)
		Celltop (Pharmacia)
		Exitop (Farmitalia Carlo Erba)
Paclitaxel	Taxol (Bristol-Myers Squibb)	Taxol (Bristol-Myers Squibb)
Vinblastine	Velban (Eli Lilly)	Velbe (Eli Lilly, Berna)
	Velsar (Adria)	

(continued)

221

Generic Name	Brand Name	
	USA (Manufacturer)	Europe (Manufacturer)
D. Agents Derived from Plants (cont.)		
Vincristine	Oncovin (Eli Lilly) Vincasar (Adria)	Oncovin (Eli Lilly, Berna) Leucid (Leo) Vincosid (Leo)
E. Hormonal Agents		
Megestrol	Megace (Bristol-Myers Squibb, Mead Johnson)	Megace (Bristol-Myers Squibb) Megeron (Neoforma) Megastat (Bristol-Myers Squibb)
Tamoxifen	Megestil (Boehringer Mannheim) Nolvadex (Zeneca, ICI) Tamofen (Bellon, Gerot, Tillotts) Tamoplex (Du Pont, Ferring, Pharmachemie)	Nolvadex (Zeneca, ICI)
F. Miscellaneous		
Acyclovir	Zovirax (Burroughs Wellcome)	Zovirax (Burroughs Wellcome) Viclovir (Abello) Virmen (Menarini) Acerpes (Hexal)

Amitriptyline	Elavil (Stuart, Hauck) Endep (Roche) Mareline (Marion)	Elavil (Merck Sharp & Dohme) Laroxyl (Roche) Lentizol (Parke Davis)
Amphotericin B	Fungizone (Bristol-Myers Squibb) Ambisone (Vestar)	Fungizone (Bristol-Myers Squibb) Ambisone (Vestar) Ampho-Moronal (Bristol-Myers Squibb, Heyden)
Calcium folinate	Leucovorin (Lederle, Burroughs Wellcome)	Lederfoline (Lederle) Citrofolin (Bracco) Elvorine (Lederle)
Ceftazidine	Fortaz (Glaxo)	Fortum (Glaxo, Cascan) Fortam (Glaxo) Ceftim (Glaxo)
Cimetidine	Tagamet	Tametin (ISF) Peptol (Horner) Gastromet (Bayropharm)
Dexamethasone	Decadron (Merck) Decameth (Foy) Millicorten (Ciba-Geigy)	Decadron (Merck Sharp & Dohme) Decasone (ICN) Maxidex (Alcon) Millicorten (Ciba-Geigy)
Diphenhydramine	Benedryl Allerdryl (ICN)	Allerdryl (Legere) Allergan (Bouty)

(continued)

Brand Name

Generic Name	USA (Manufacturer)	Europe (Manufacturer)
F. Miscellaneous (cont.)		
Epogen	Epogen (Amgen)	Exprex (Cilag, Ortho)
	Procrit (Amgen, Ortho)	Erypo (Janssen)
		Globuren (Dompe Biotec)
Famcyclovir	Famvir (SmithKline Beecham)	Famvir (SmithKline Beecham)
Filgrastim (G-CSF)	Neupogen (Amgen)	Neupogen (Amgen, Dompe (Amgen, Dompe
		Granulokine (Roche)
Gentamycin	Garamycin	Garamycin (Essex, Scherineg-Plough)
	Gentak (Akorn)	Gentamin (Medix)
Granisetron	Kytril (SmithKline Beecham)	Kytril (SmithKline Beecham)
Hydrocortisone	Solu-Cortef (Upjohn)	Solu-Cortef (Upjohn)
Kaopectate	Kaopectate (Upjohn)	Kaopectate (Upjohn)
Lorazepam	Ativan (Wyeth)	Ativan (Wyeth)
Metoclopramide	Reglan (Robins)	Reglan (Wyeth-Ayerst, Delagrange)
	Clopromate (Purdue Frederick)	Metoclamid (Hexal)
	Octamide (Adria)	Emetid (Virbac)
Metronidazole	Flagyl (Searle)	Flagyl (Specia, Rhone-Paulenc, Farmitalia Carlo Erba)
	Elyzol (Dumex)	
	Metrizol (Cyanamid)	

Ondansetron	Zofran (Glaxo, Cerenex)	Zofran (Glaxo) Zophren (Glaxo) Finox (Findiet)
Piperacillin	Pipracil (Lederle)	Pipracil (Lederle) Pipril (Lederle) Avocin (Cyanamid)
Ranitidine	Zantac (Glaxo)	Zantac (Glaxo) Azantic (Glaxo) Coralen (Alter)
Sargramostim (GM-CSF)	Leukine (Immunex) Profine (Hoechst)	Interberin (Behring)
Ticarcillin	Ticar (SmithKline Beecham) Timentin (SmithKline Beecham)	Ticar (SmithKline Beecham) Claventin (SmithKline Beecham) Aerugipen (Beecham-Wulfing)
Tobramycin	Tobrex (Alcon)	Tobrex (Alcon) Tobralex (Alcon) Bruamycin (Labatec)
Vancomycin	Vancocin (Lilly) Vancor (Adria) Lyphocin (Lyphomed)	Vancocin (Eli Lilly, Berna) Vancocina (Lilly) Vancocine (Lilly)

SELECTED READING

DuBois D, DuBois EF: A formula to estimate the approximate surface area if height and weight are known. *Arch Intern Med* 1916; 17:863-871.

Haycock GB, Schwartz GJ, Wisotsky DH: Geometric method for measuring body surface area: A height-weight formula validated in infants, children, and adults. *J Pediatr* 1978; 93:62-66.

Karnofsky DA, Abelmann WH, Craver LF, et al: The use of the nitrogen mustards in the palliative treatment of carcinoma. *Cancer* 1948; 1:634-656.

Mostellar RD: Simplified calculation of body-surface area. N *Engl J Med* 1987; 317:1098.

Oken MM, Creech RH, Tormey DC, et al: Toxicity and response criteria of the Eastern Cooperative Oncology Group. *Am J Clin Oncol* 1982; 5:649-655.

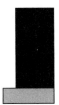

INDEX

Page numbers followed by f indicate figures; t, tables.